Caring

People of the Clouds

AGING AND DEMENTIA IN OAXACA

JONATHAN YAHALOM

FOREWORD BY XAVIER E. CAGIGAS

UNIVERSITY OF OKLAHOMA PRESS : NORMAN

Library of Congress Cataloging-in-Publication Data

Names: Yahalom, Jonathan, 1985– author.
Title: Caring for the people of the clouds : aging and dementia in Oaxaca / Jonathan
    Yahalom; foreword by Xavier E. Cagigas.
Description: Norman : University of Oklahoma Press, [2019] | Includes bibliographical
    references and index.
Identifiers: LCCN 2018033739| ISBN 978-0-8061-6268-3 (hardcover : alk. paper) |
    ISBN 978-0-8061-6304-8 (pbk.   )
Subjects: LCSH: Dementia—Mexico—Oaxaca (State) | Aging—Mexico—Oaxaca
    (State) | Caregivers.
Classification: LCC RC521 .Y34 2019 | DDC 616.8/310097274—dc23
LC record available at https://lccn.loc.gov/2018033739

For my family

Contents

Illustrations

TABLE

CHARTS

Foreword

XAVIER E. CAGIGAS

Those who know nothing of foreign languages know nothing of their own.
—Johann Wolfgang von Goethe

As a young boy I came to believe that certain books had a habit of choosing me as their reader, rather than my choosing to read them. Subsequently during my undergraduate years, I came across a collection of letters between Carl Gustav Jung and Wolfgang Pauli entitled *Atom and Archetype*, in which Jung and Pauli elaborated on their independently derived notions of synchronicity from their respective perspectives as psychologist and physicist. I was simultaneously introduced to the magical realism of Jorge Luis Borges and Gabriel García-Márquez, which only fed my intellectual curiosity and childhood observation that the universe seems to conspire in bringing about intellectual perspectives that challenge conventional thinking in fresh and often unexpected ways. The book you are about to read is yet another such occurrence in my life, borne of my stumbling into an academic research talk at the UCLA Chicano Studies Research Center entitled "Caregiving in Oaxaca: Social Perspectives on Aging and Dementia," followed by a dialogue with Jonathan Yahalom that seemed to weave together various epochs within my own life: research on the subjective experience of Alzheimer's disease, facilitating caregiver support groups, founding a clinical service and training program at UCLA that is dedicated to bilingual assessment in cultural neuropsychology with Latinos, having a Oaxacan *ahijada* (goddaughter), and my academic penchant for trying to reconcile what Vygotsky once dubbed the "crisis in psychology."

Caring for the People of the Clouds harkens back to themes of Wilhelm Wundt's "second psychology," or *Völkerpsychologie*, the vibrant folk psychology of the people as a complement to the sterile brass instrument psychology of his time. It is situated within the tradition of pioneering cultural psychologist and neuropsychologist Alexander Luria's expedition to rural Uzbekistan during which he attempted to capture rapid socio-historical and cultural changes in cognition. It echoes the renowned neurologist Oliver Sacks's eloquent exposition of the case study illustrating the complementary nature of what Luria himself referred to as classical and romantic science. In essence, Yahalom's book evokes memories of a scholarly tradition that many have come to overlook—one that embraces a phenomenological approach to scientific inquiry and that is guided by qualitative observation and detailed description rather than mere quantitative execution and dissection.

Through what Roy D'Andrade coined as cognitive ethnography, this book introduces a novel clinical sensitivity that makes apparent both the epistemological and pragmatic challenges posed by the meeting of two different worlds: the neurobiological undergirding of scientific explanations for dementia on the one hand, and the lived collectivist experience of forgetting in the people of Teotitlán on the other. Indeed, the concept of *mestizaje* seems rather apropos in describing how Yahalom masterfully weaves together seemingly disparate threads of experience to form a new understanding of what dementia has come to signify semiotically in a type of nomothetic/idiographic dialectic. He artfully resists the impulse to adopt a more hegemonic narrative, and instead presents an alternative to the mere intellectual colonization of what could be perceived as a reified and exotic cultural curiosity. Specifically, Yahalom adopts a stance of cultural humility that both clarifies and challenges the broader status quo's understanding of embodied dementia. This book, then, is particularly timely given renewed interest throughout academic medicine in developing cultural and linguistic competence in the delivery of clinical services to a widening, diverse, and aging demographic, while at the same time recognizing the imminent need to improve empirical studies through more equitable and proportional inclusion of historically underrepresented populations in research.

The value of Yahalom's book, however, clearly reaches beyond his helping to articulate voices that have historically gone unheard; I believe that the sophistication of his narrative also speaks to the current state of the crisis in psychology.

He embraces the primacy of human experience riddled with all its idiosyncratic complexity, thereby elevating the level of scholarly discourse beyond a mere reductionist frame toward the phenomenological fabric of true understanding.

This book satisfies both the humanistic and donnish reader by interlacing emotive points of dialogue from lived experience with the fundamental scientific assumptions that subserve our understanding of how dementia manifests in the quotidian lives of people and their communities. Its fresh ideas articulate a type of zeitgeist whose ripples are found in the fields of cultural neuroscience, neuroanthropology, and my own cultural neuropsychology. Indeed, this intimate focus on cultural practices, meaningfully distributed and rooted throughout people's actual lived experiences, serves as a window into the workings of the human mind and brain, which is the cornerstone of cultural neuropsychology.

I therefore ask you, the reader, to entertain the possibility that perhaps this book has chosen you for a reason, in much the same way it has chosen me. As a consequence, my understanding of dementia and what constitutes its appropriate unit of analysis has undergone a healthy revision within these pages, and my walk with the clouds has given way to a clearer understanding of the path I tread as clinician, scientist, and human being.

Preface

I am neither an anthropologist nor a scholar of Mexican studies. I am a clinical psychologist. And it was working within my own field—striving to understand people in order to reduce their suffering—that sparked my engagement with these other disciplines.

This book is an ethnography about family caregiving for elders with dementia in a rural—"indigenous"—Oaxacan community. Scare quotes are deliberate; I learned from my readings in anthropology that such categorizations are as helpful as they are problematic, as descriptive as they are misleading.[1] I study the Oaxacan social world as a means to contextualize caregiving and, analogously, analyze caregiving as a prism to understand what is at stake for individuals living in Oaxaca. In its broadest sense, then, this book explores the social construction of caregiving for elders living with dementia in this community.

I anticipate that among my colleagues in psychology—working within a discipline that defines itself as producing objective, empirical knowledge of human experience—some might handle a book on social construction with a certain uneasiness. Readers might dismiss this project for not being sufficiently scientific. But in these initial pages I want to frame why this approach arose from directly engaging with psychology as an empirical science.

During my clinical training, I sought readings outside psychology when I tried to think seriously about cultural competence: what it means to be effective in working with people of different backgrounds. Providing talk therapy to help people grow and overcome life difficulties showed that this this type of competence was not just an auxiliary to clinical practice, but one that directly concerned how individuals are able to develop confidence to disclose sensitive information about their lives. Psychotherapy, after all, is premised on talking honestly, and it is only through encouraging individuals to be honest about the specific ways they experience the world that one can realize the fruits of this endeavor. I was fortunate to have been trained by a number of thoughtful and skilled supervisors—all of whom, in varying ways, taught by example about how to work with the concrete, specific details of people's experience. Working this way seemed to imbue clinical practice with therapeutic valence, and my own experience as a clinician with personal meaning.

But I also began to realize that the good therapy I was taught seemed different from the best practices I studied. In the literature on cultural competence, I began to see how gaining knowledge of essentialized summaries of "culture" differed from the ways my supervisors effectively taught clinical sensitivity. "Asian Americans prefer a more directed therapy," I read, "whereas Latin Americans prefer one that incorporates the family." Such statements *might* prove true, but assuming them prior to learning from patients robs people of their agency—and therapists of genuine understanding. This not only goes against what I learned in my training, but also undermines the fluidity that defines the first of the American Psychological Association's *Multicultural Guidelines*: "to recognize and understand that identity and self-definition are fluid and complex and that the interaction between the two is dynamic" (APA, 2017, p. 6).[2]

How my field practices cultural competence as a matter of fluidity seemed different from how it tends to define culture as a static set of characteristics. Clinical training taught that culture is not something one can operationalize and master, but something that unsettles knowledge and disrupts assumptions. Culture in this sense approximates what philosopher Emmanuel Levinas (1969/1992) describes as "otherness" or "alterity"—the different characteristics of another person that are, *by their nature of being different*, incapable of being fully known. Conceptual knowledge erases difference—or, to put it oppositely, difference ruptures knowledge. Levinas's point is that once we purport to know and master understanding of another person's difference, the act of knowing levels those characteristics into our own conceptual framework, thereby erasing what marks that person as different to begin with.

This means that while we might do well—indeed *ought*—to familiarize ourselves with other ways of life and other cultures, this does not mean we have "mastered" anything. Again quoting the APA's *Multicultural Guidelines:* "cultural competence does not refer to a process that ends simply because the psychologist is deemed competent. Rather, cultural competence incorporates the role of cultural humility whereby cultural competence is considered a lifelong process of reflection and commitment" (p. 8; see also Tervalon & Murray-Garcia, 1998).

Anthropology helps provide a theory (social constructionism) and method (ethnography) of studying culture that guard against assuming that such studies produce anything resembling mastery. In its broadest sense, the ethnographic method is a process of studying another's lifestyle. It is related to qualitative forms of inquiry that invite participants to share aspects of their lived experience without forced-choice answers that tend to conceal details. Like APA's notion of cultural competence, and psychotherapeutic practice in general, ethnography invites people to speak and, when they do so, highlights researchers' humbling experience as they listen. "Ethnography is valued not only as a means to bear witness to people's lived experience," write Wilkinson and Kleinman (2016), "but also for its potential to discomfit and unsettle the researcher" (p. 157). It gives authority to local knowledge and other people's experiences, which is why Clifford and Marcus (1986) rather positively refer to ethnographies as "true fictions," an oxymoron that reminds researchers that they are striving for the truth about human experience while recognizing that the truth is always partial, in flux, and contested (pp. 7–8). This is the truth inherent to ethnography, but also to the nature of cultural knowledge as well.

Social constructionism (and pragmatism, its epistemological cousin that I adopt in this book) provide an accompanying approach to conceptualize knowledge that is nonauthoritative and decentering. The idea is that some of the basic things we hold to be true are shaped by specific social arrangements. So, truth is contingent, and what we perceive as true could conceivably be different, depending on surrounding social circumstances.[3]

Not surprisingly, the majority in scientific disciplines, psychology included, view this approach with considerable suspicion. It is not only unfair to personal experience but also dangerous to claim, for example, that all approaches to treating illness are equal when there is unequivocal evidence that some treatments are more effective than others. I agree. Yet by the same token, the stance that some forms of thoughts, beliefs, and perspectives of the world are more truthful than others does harm toward facilitating a genuine account of culture. At best, it advances cultural knowledge that is implicitly skeptical and unintentionally belittling. A constructionist approach provides one solution. As I use it, it offers an epistemological framework to studying cultural truths that, to borrow a term from the phenomenological tradition, "brackets" the assumption that some forms of knowledge are more accurate than others. Anthropologists are on the right track in saying that this epistemological shift is required when aiming to learn something new about another way of life. Yet I also appeal to the phenomenological bracket because I purposefully avoid making any generalized claim like "all truths are constructed." Such generalizations are not only counter to what I personally hold about certain facts in the world, but also distract from the function this epistemology serves in studying other people's experience. Instead, I consider how some of the things I consider true about aging, mental health, and related forms of care are expressions of my own cultural outlook. I adopt this perspective as a researcher and clinician who wants to unsettle his own conviction about truth in order to remain open to learning about the ones other people live by.

Around the same time as I developed interest in anthropology, I began researching Alzheimer's disease because I considered myself (and broader U.S. culture) limited in confronting issues pertaining to death and dying. I began to consider not only how death seemed absent in everyday experience, but also how old age appeared to be something one succumbs to—instead of a life stage imbued with meaning. As historian Thomas Cole (1992) writes of the impact of this sentiment, "a culture that denies death as an integral part of life . . . must also deny old age as an integral part of life" (p. 141). I reasoned that studying Alzheimer's as one form of death and dying would deepen my own personal understanding and professionally challenge this social outlook.

I initially turned to neuroscience and became fascinated by alarming statistics and promising technologies—all indicating the prominence of Alzheimer's today. It is one of the more recognized illnesses in the United States, commonly referred to as an "epidemic," and increasingly prevalent as the population ages. The disease accounts for the large majority of cases pertaining to age-related dementia, with researchers positing that underlying neuropathology (plaques and tangles) lead to progressive cognitive decline. And while Alzheimer's has been a household term since the 1980s, cases will not only rise owing to population gains, but also by the introduction of new screening technologies that can predict illness prior to the onset of symptoms. The presence of these technologies now makes diagnosis more common than ever.[4]

Yet for all the curiosity stimulated from within my own discipline, I soon realized that a narrow focus on neuroscience and related technology would not provide the answers I was looking for. I wanted to know how Alzheimer's is experienced within our tendencies to fear, and efforts to prevent, death. As such, I knew I had to consider the actual way Alzheimer's is lived, not just epidemiological and neurological models abstracted from it. Novelist Jonathan Franzen (2007) describes a similar sentiment when he writes of his reaction to his father's decline.

> I can see my reluctance to apply the term "Alzheimer's" to my father as a way of protecting the specificity of Earl Franzen from the generality of a nameable condition. Conditions have symptoms; symptoms point to the organic basis of everything we are. They point to the brain as meat. And, where I ought to recognize that, yes, the brain is meat, I seem instead to maintain a blind spot across which I then interpolate stories that emphasize the more soul-like aspects of the self. Seeing my afflicted father as a set of organic symptoms would . . . reduce our beloved personalities to finite sets of neurochemical coordinates. Who wants a story of life like that? (pp. 19–20)

Whatever story one chooses, Franzen's powerful words remind us that there exists an additional story that stands apart from neuroscience itself. It is a story not about neurological failure, but the way life exists in the context of that failure. It is a story about the lived experience of Alzheimer's, how persons continue to function, respond, and die within the parameters of illness.

I experienced this sentiment as an injunction to define the direction of my clinical training. I sought knowledge by working at different geriatric hospital units where I had the opportunity to observe and participate in the diagnosis, treatment, and reintegration of elders. I read a wide variety of clinical texts, but was most impacted by Oliver Sacks's (1998) beautifully simple description of human agency behind illness. He writes that our understanding of illness must extend beyond pathology because symptoms always involve "a reaction . . . to restore, to replace, to compensate for and to preserve [a person's] identity" (p. 6). Here was a statement that at once acknowledged the devastating course of neuropathology, but also pointed to the necessity of situating it in the surrounding human world.

In this way, I came to view Alzheimer's as vital to study not just as an objective process that occurs in one's brain, but also as an expression of human will.[5]

Yet I soon realized that the questions I was interested in asking would not be fully answered by books and training in my tradition. I needed to supplement my clinical curriculum, to turn to disciplines that extended beyond the realm of psychology to understand the social factors that contextualize psychological ones. I decided to research caregivers to better appreciate these factors, and the way in which the care they provided embodied the social life I wanted to understand. Further, I reasoned that conducting a study in another cultural setting would require me to continually question basic ideas about death, dying, and illness, and help provide contrastive light on these taken-for-granted concepts from my own background. As I will describe in the following pages, Oaxaca seemed an ideal place to carry out such an investigation, and anthropology came to provide the relevant framework I need to obtain the answers I sought.

Inasmuch as I ask for openness among my colleagues in psychology to consider how this approach enriches our knowledge and practice, I ask for similar consideration among anthropologists and researchers in Mexican studies as a guest to their fields. Beyond clinical psychology, in this book I hope to contribute to contemporary research on Mexico and the anthropology of care, and perhaps to provide a different approach to conceptualizing relevant themes. I do my best to understand these fields with the same rigor as I practice clinically but, like working across cultures, I recognize that the rewards of interdisciplinarity are accompanied by its challenges. I hope the endeavor merits the effort.

Acknowledgments

The lessons drawn from this study parallel my experience conducting it. That the progress one makes is only realized through the support of those generous to offer it, that life meaning and purpose and fulfillment are not individual accomplishments that somehow render a person unique, but shared projects that bring people in various ways together. Between the lines written in this book stand the numerous stories of the people who made it possible.

When I pause to think about it, the origins of this project go back to my initial desire to become a psychologist. Years ago, in northern California and on the way to wine country with my mother and stepfather, I debated whether to leave my job at Google to pursue a new career in psychology. My parents embodied the care that informed so much of my sensibility found in this book: they listened, they understood, and they responded with love and support. And so, months later, I announced to my father, Aba, at our favorite San Francisco restaurant, the Mona Lisa, that I would be moving to Pittsburgh for my studies. We celebrated with a bottle of wine that would only be opened when I finished my new vocational path. Now this book marks yet another step toward the pursuit of that dream, the realization of why those initial conversations mattered so much back then. I am beyond indebted to *all* my parents—my mom, Aba,

Glen, Sylvia, and Luisa—for their understanding, support, and love. May we keep having more wine to open and more occasions to celebrate—*l'chaim!*

I am equally blessed for my little brother, Joshie, whose joy inspires and whose companionship has always made life richer. My aunt and uncle, Nomi Shragai and Charlie Morris, have been bastions of support, especially during my time in Oaxaca through our "writing club." This is but one instance of so many other projects they have helped me accomplish through their guidance and encouragement. And also, thank you to the rest of my family, whose encouragement and interest helped provide further motivation to see this project to completion.

Research for this book has always been inspired by the memory of Tommy Sage Hand, whose life-affirming jest and philosophically inspired compassion have continued to guide me. If—to recall the conversations we shared—we never stop growing and learning, if we always keep pressing forward, these subsequent pages have been written alongside the spirit of this companion I was so fortunate to call my friend.

I am well aware that this book on Oaxaca is written by someone from outside the community. Aside from the benefits of perspective and problems of presumption in endeavoring such a project, my experience partnering with, growing from, and relying on others has all been premised on a type of hospitality that continues to inspire me years later. This was never just an "academic" study but a deeply personal work, and I am incredibly grateful to so many individuals for opening their homes, sharing their stories, and developing new friendships with me. During my fieldwork I was a guest scholar under Dra. Paola Sesia at *Centro de Investigaciones y Estudios Superiores en Antropología Social* (CIESAS), where I not only developed my anthropological gaze but was also taught the true, collaborative spirit of academic inquiry. Additionally, my residency at *La Biblioteca de Investigación Juan de Córdova* provided an inspiring space to reflect and write. Thanks to Michael Swanton for his hospitality and enthusiasm to document what I came to learn. *También, yo quisiera agradecer a las empleados y amigos de la biblioteca, especialmente a Janet Chavez Santiago, mi buena amiga y maestra de Zapoteco. Muchísimas gracias por todos los años de aprendizaje y por tu amistad.*

This project would not have been possible without the help I received in Teotitlán del Valle. I would like to express deep gratitude to Taurino Alexandro "Alex" Mendoza Martínez and family for so warmly welcoming me into their home and helping establish local contacts. As this book will come to document, Alex is in many ways the hero of this story, and I am sincerely grateful for his willingness to take it on as his own personal endeavor. *Además yo quisiera mencionar a Domingo Gutierrez Mendoza quien me ha ayudado entender las experiencias de los adultos mayores en Teotitlán, Cristy Martinez Molina y familia, el municipio de Teotitlán, y el resto de mis amigos teotitecos. Finalmente, quisiera dar las gracias a todas las personas que me ayudaron a hacer posible este proyecto—especialmente cada familia con todo el cariño quien me dieron en su casa. Espero que este proyecto haga justicia para contar su historia. ¡Xtiusen yubtuu!*

Studying clinical and theoretical psychology at Duquesne University has been a privilege. Leswin Laubscher has led by example in demonstrating what passionate scholarship looks like; I'm fortunate to call him a mentor, advocate, and friend. Elizabeth Fein has continued to provide guidance and support from the beginning of my fieldwork to its very end. Roger Brooke provided the encouragement to pursue an interdisciplinary project on aging. James Swindal has been generous in supporting this project through the Dissertation Fellowship on behalf of the McAnulty College and Graduate School of Liberal Arts. The Gumberg Library staff was supportive and patient through helping track down obscure books and articles. Thank you also to Marilyn Henline and Linda "the Boss" Pasqualino. And, lastly, thanks to fellow graduate students and friends who motivated me in school and outside: Teal Fitzpatrick, Chris McCann, Denise Mahone, Rachel Gotleib, and Katie Wagner.

While this book is largely focused on nonclinical work, it was inspired by the everyday lessons I learned while engaged in therapeutic practice. I am especially appreciative for the numerous clinical supervisors I have been so fortunate to train under. Thank you especially to Jessie Goicoechea, Bruce Fink, Roger Brooke, Lynn Northrop, and Greg Serpa.

The final phases of writing occurred through a generous visiting-scholar position offered by UCLA's Chicano Studies Research Center. Thank you to Rebecca Epstein and the rest of CSRC faculty and staff for extending such hospitality and support. Within this inspiring community, I am thankful for the opportunity to participate in and be intellectually stimulated by the Mind Medicine and Culture seminars held by the Anthropology Department. Thank you also to Xavier E. Cagigas, who supported this project with kind generosity and academic hospitality.

Thank you to numerous individuals at the University of Oklahoma Press. I am especially appreciative of Alessandra Tamulevich for ongoing guidance and being the first person to see potential in this project prior to it coming to fruition; Walt Evans for detailed editorial help; and Stephanie Evans, Amy Hernandez, and the rest of the Press staff who helped promote, complete, and improve the quality of this book.

Lastly, I would like to sincerely thank the friends and colleagues who have, in so many ways, significantly contributed to my work. Many thanks to Andy Moore for editorial mastery in helping sharpen the manuscript and coyote-inspired friendship. Thank you to Bonnie Kaiser and Jo Weaver for collaboration and guidance in developing a key chapter of this book. In Oaxaca, my gratitude extends to Sebastian Pillitteri, Sophie Langridge, Eric Fanghanel, Andrea Gilly, Kat Black, Nan "Lola" Newell, Holly Worthen, Whitney Duncan, Peter Guarnaccia, Karen Rasmussen, Leidy Jarquin Saucedo, Eduardo Sánchez García, Leticia Gomez Salinas, Juan Vera, and Bricia Irene Cruz Matus for friendship, shared interest in my project, and help understanding local life. From Pittsburgh, thanks to Kryn and Kiara Sausedo, Ad and Jill Yeomans, Lindsay Reed, and Erika Beras for ongoing encouragement throughout graduate school and beyond. From the VA, thank you to Jess Alva, Ryan Brewster, Ahoo Karimian, Barbara Wettstein, Deniz Ahmadinia, Ippy Kalofonos, and Noah Bussell. From California, with both old and new people in my life, my deep gratitude extends to Michelle Nermon, Ben Hamlin, Xander Marin, the Court Family (Colin, Kelly, Theo, and Millie), Justin Christianson, Adam Wright, AJ and Shooter Bisciglia, Lauren Lindsay, Drew Grabiner, Emma Knickerbocker, Jenna Van Slyke, Yasmine Pollak, and numerous other friends and family who provide the zest of what makes life meaningful, and whose presence continues to enrich it day after day.

Caring for the
People
of the
Clouds

Introduction

An old woman stood on the side of the road. Her wrinkled face spoke to a certain endurance; her stillness seemed to protest the oncoming rush of traffic. The road leaving Oaxaca City radiated with intense August heat. Her dark-gray hair, woven in braids, hung over an apron that was threadbare and embroidered with multicolored flowers. She was alone beside a burlap grocery bag, returning home from what appeared to be the culmination of morning errands.

This was one of the first images I remember from a year of research in Oaxaca. I had traveled to this region of southern Mexico to conduct an investigation on what I then could only vaguely state was interest in caregiving for dementia. I wanted to know how aging and caregiving for elders might differ across time and place. In the process, I came to learn about how those differences speak to the profound ways culture dynamically constitutes human experience, and to the importance of attending to this dynamic nature while working with other people.

The woman on the side of the road was memorable for putting into focus an image of aging from the outside—testifying to elders' autonomy and empowerment, and to the juxtaposition of age-old traditions against modern social changes. But this early experience was also important for exposing me to a complementary, more nuanced image from inside private doors. I was heading to Teotitlán del Valle (hereafter Teotitlán), a small Zapotec-speaking community a forty-minute drive away from Oaxaca City, the state capital.

Many foreigners visit Teotitlán as part of the standard tourist circuit, but on this day I was traveling to meet "Alex," a 25-year-old local with whom I had corresponded via email, months prior. Alex greeted me at his home in his airy courtyard, with an infant resting in his arms. He and his wife were in the process of dying wool, and the scene called my attention to the bold colors surrounding the space. Dyed skeins hung from one wall and on others were commanding *tapetes* (rugs) for which Teotitlán has earned its fame. In the kitchen were his mother and paternal grandmother preparing *chorizo* in anticipation of my visit. Both women were wearing an apron similar to the one I had noticed earlier, but my interaction with them was limited while they worked in the kitchen. They spoke to each other in Zapotec, one of Oaxaca's sixteen indigenous languages that appeared more related to eastern languages than romantic ones. Through the course of my visit, Alex and I exchanged personal stories of our mutual experiences in California (where I grew up and he had worked and studied), ate lunch with his family, and eventually found time to discuss the nature of my project. Across a wooden dining room table and below a towering muted TV, he translated the conversation in Zapotec for his grandmother and in a combination of English and Spanish for me. At one point Alex looked over at his sleeping infant and told me that he hoped to teach his son Zapotec to communicate with family elders and the community, but also English should he live and work in California.

In retrospect, these two contrastive scenes—the woman on public streets and the family in Alex's home—put into focus a conceptual disparity that would constitute the object of my research in Oaxaca. It highlighted poles between how aging might be represented through an image of enduring mettle, and a much more complicated scene marked by the confluence of different languages, temporal horizons, and generational difference. The first points to how old age is viewed nonproblematically, how even Oaxacans tend to celebrate elders for their enduring vitality and normative authority. The second reveals a more complicated view of aging and its constitution within broad social transformations and subsequent uncertainties—including tensions—that manifest in daily life, what Jennifer Cole and Deborah Durham (2007) call the "intimate politics of globalization" (p. 19). Such intimacy refers to the ways in which global shifts in capital, resources, and power are experienced and responded to in caring for elders, and how specific households within local communities negotiate and adapt to such change to meet elders' needs. Nearly all that I witnessed in Alex's home was steeped in this dynamic between age and change—and notably suffused in a degree of care that marked his response: care for the well-being of his family; care to maintain local identity in the context of global influence; and care to facilitate intergenerational connection while anticipating its fissure by different languages, geographies, and customs. As others before me, I came to appreciate how age itself—and care for the aged—is a prism for this larger social dynamic. This book sheds light on this process, exploring how caring for elders and the concomitant injunction to maintain a sense of cohesion manifest in the context of broader social change.

~

The Zapotec people of Teotitlán are principally Catholic, but the pre-Hispanic religious meaning of their name provides clues to local notions about aging. The word "Zapotec" simultaneously refers to a cultural group and its language. It is a literal derivation from Nahuatl, the language of the Aztec kingdom, and means "people of the *zapote*," a species of local fruit. But locally they call themselves *bènizàa*, a Zapotec word that means "people of the clouds." This references a former practice of worshipping royal ancestors who, after passing, were believed to transform into divine spirits—clouds—that resided in the sky to protect the community (J. Marcus & Flannery, 1996, p. 20).[1] These ancestors were termed "old people of the clouds," giving rise to the local meaning of the word Zapotec. This historical concept continues to endure, and provides what is perhaps the earliest vestige of how elders today are revered for their embodiment of tradition and authority about how to practice it.

In a setting like Teotitlán, it is instructive that elders are so intimately tied to local representations of tradition because both tradition and old age are heralded as anchors to local identity. The Zapotec word for elders, *bengul*, is a term that connotes authority and prestige and refers to one's accumulated life experience and wisdom. These individuals are recognized within the community as reference points for how to properly practice local tradition. Typically, elders are called upon at weddings to give the first piece of advice to married couples, are the first to enter and sit closest to the altar room to pay respect to family ancestors, have the last word to settle disputes, and are asked to make other judgments about whether communal practices adhere to local tradition. These practices help maintain social cohesion. Yet insofar as elders are represented as a bulwark of tradition, this association also implies vulnerability; community members must practice tradition to keep it alive; and many elders lead different lifestyles with new physical constraints that impart dependency. Indeed, in

Teotitlán today, both the meaning of old age and the practices of tradition are shifting in the context of broader social change. Precisely because of their susceptibly to change and loss, elders and tradition must be cared for—and it is through acts of care that the value of old age and tradition is expressed.

~

I arrived in Oaxaca not as an anthropologist but as a clinical psychologist with general interest in caring practices. Like others in the mental health fields, my therapeutic sensibility was defined by caring for those in need. Yet, ironically, for disciplines premised on care, I found psychology and related practices overlooking something essential about the overall nature of care. Research about ways certain conditions necessitate care, characteristics of competent care, and why some interventions work over others generates important and useful knowledge. But in the treatment manuals and research articles that dominate my discipline, something about the nature of care seemed lost. Psychology has become so focused on operationalizing "care" that, though well intentioned, it often attempts to lay out definitions and techniques before exploring sensibilities and experiences. And this, replacing experience for generalization, overlooks a major reason people seek help: to feel truly seen and heard, to find healing in this relational space, and to develop subsequent connection to the surrounding world.

For clinicians, this return to sensibility and experience brings the human-ity back into its appropriate place within the practice of therapy. How much more is provided when we move from describing a person as an "Alzheimer's caregiver" to understanding the experience of having a deep relationship with a progressively forgetful person who no longer responds when he is called "Dad."[2] It is through attending to this detailed, lived experience that the nature of care is embodied, which is why Mol, Moser, and Pols (2010) caution that, if we allow operationalized terms to replace subjective, lived experience, then what we call "caregiving" will be very different than care itself. In their words, "[An abstract, operationalized approach to understanding caregiving] threatens to take the heart out of care—and along with this not just its kindness but also its effectiveness, its tenacity and its strength" (p. 7).

Caring for the People of the Clouds is a response to this threat, and is an illustra-tion of therapeutic hearing about caring practices that remains anchored in a sensibility of care. It is a study of the detailed, lived experience of caregiving for dependent elders living with dementia in Teotitlán, with attention to how this experience is constituted within and responsive to the surrounding social world. This site proves a rich location for this endeavor, as everyday experience is riddled with issues concerning social change and concomitant questions about how to maintain social cohesion in its context. Among many other studies in Mexico, past research has explored the way the aging body is negotiated between Mexican stereotypes about family loyalty and contrasting ones about *machismo* (Wentzell, 2013), how social reproductive strategies inherent to motherhood adapt in the face of global migration (Smith-Oka, 2013), and how, specifically in Oaxaca, there exists an underlying "psychological modernization" project that promotes a different, globalized vision of selfhood that contests local understandings (Duncan, 2018). This book contributes to these studies by exploring the social relations that arise in the context of caregiving for elders with dementia in Oaxaca and, in so doing, provides insight into how these relations embody the negotiation of broader social dynamics on a daily level. This book also draws on the pioneering and illuminating set of research conducted specifically in Teotitlán, helping put into focus how local identity is transnationally stretched across borders (Stephen, 2007; Wood, 2008), gender dynamics as Teotitlán economically transforms (Stephen, 2005), as well as other general information pertinent to local culture, economics, and lifestyle.[3] Moreover, as a book on caregiving, it dialogues with what Buch (2015) has termed the "veritable explosion" of research on the anthropology of care that explores what it means to care in the context of social change (L. Cohen, 1998; Ticktin, 2011), the nature of caregiving in settings marked by social absences owing to migration (Parreñas, 2005; Yarris, 2017), and the economies of care as responsibilities circulate across transnational spaces (Abrego, 2014; Baldassar & Merla, 2013; Leinaweaver, 2005; Parreñas, 2015). Drawing on these insights, this book analyzes caregiving as a means to understand more about the social dimensions of care itself. In attending to relevant cultural values that inform and sustain local caregiving practices—and the way those values are affirmed and regenerated in the process—this book offers a lesson about why attending to the concrete, nuanced details of caregiving is instructive for the anthropology of care and for the clinical sciences that aim to practice it.

LOCATING OAXACA IN A GLOBALIZED WORLD

Perhaps the surest way to acquaint oneself with Oaxaca is to first take note of its cheese. Local *quesillo* is produced in a continuous, inch-thick strip that coils to form a ball, sometimes so massive that it exceeds a foot in diameter. In markets vendors stand behind their large globes, waiting for a customer's order, and then deftly unravel the round morass. "Oaxaca is like its cheese," people are apt to say, "so complicated that even *it* is tied in knots."

Oaxaca is so entwined through being situated within a very specific defini-tion of local identity while being stretched through engagement with global influences. To understand Oaxaca and appreciate what is at stake in Oaxacan social life, one must attend to this dynamic and the way it situates a unique imperative to maintain local identity and social cohesion.

Part of Oaxaca's identity can be understood through its dramatic regional geography. Oaxaca is composed of two mountain ranges—the Sierra Norte and Sierra Sur—whose rugged terrain even today continues to render access to many regions difficult, with serpentine roads that test the limits of most people's stomachs. While the state's total area is about two-thirds the size of Pennsylvania—and just less than 5 percent of Mexico's total landmass—Oaxaca has many microclimates and is recognized for being a biological "hotspot" with a rich array of plant and animal life that has attracted researchers and tourists alike (Cummings, 2002).[4] Analogously, Oaxacan communities have developed distinct cultural identities, despite having been annexed by different empires and nations and situated within various economies throughout their histories.[5]

This means that, across the state, identity is not based upon broad ethnic or national categories—not terms like *Zapoteco* or even *Oaxaqueño*—but rather through *comunidad*, a much more specific notion that points to the precise com-munity (sometimes populated by fewer than one hundred persons) in which individuals grew up. Hence, when presented with the question about "what" or "who" a person is, the people of Teotitlán first and foremost consider themselves "Teotitecos"—people from Teotitlán—prior to any other ethnic, state, or national specification.[6] This sense of hyperlocal identity to the 5,500-member community is, in part, embodied through language practices. Although Teotitlán is one of Oaxaca's many Zapotec-speaking communities, nearly all of Oaxaca's rural communities have their own dialect and use language to differentiate themselves from neighbors. Teotitecos readily distinguish their language from the Zapotec spoken in places like Tlacolula (seven miles away) and Mitla (fifteen miles away), and experience serious difficulty understanding the Zapotec spoken in the surrounding mountains and other state regions.[7] In significant ways, language is not only a signifier for indigenous identity, but more importantly a means for establishing a sense of belonging to a specific community.

It is commonly claimed that Oaxaca is home to sixteen indigenous groups and respective languages. Oaxaca features 34 percent of Mexico's total indigenous-speaking populations, making it the state with the highest proportion of indig-enous-language speakers (INEGI, 2014). As a group of community-specific languages, Zapotec is the most popular non-Spanish language, with 450,000 speakers across the state. Oaxaca also features 23 percent of Mexico's *municip-ios* (municipal governments), 73 percent of which are governed according to their own *usos y costumbres* (customs and traditions). And yet, like language practices, these governments also reveal Oaxaca's hyperlocal forms of identity. The majority of municipios create their own laws and legal practices that further define unique community-specific characteristics. For example, municipios are the governing bodies that manage *tequio* and *cargo* systems, forms of voluntary labor required of citizens. Cargos are so important for the maintenance of local identity that Jeffrey Cohen (2004) calls them the contemporary "heart of village politics" for being a lifeline for its preservation (p. 14).[8] In Teotitlán today, each household is expected to provide at least one individual to carry out successive one-, two-, or three-year terms of unpaid cargo service.[9] Collecting bus fares, managing land allocation, serving as the municipal president, as well as residing over judicial and religious responsibilities all help promote local governance and ensure that local celebrations and traditions are upheld. And, in so doing, this system also bolsters the social status of community elders: first, it allots the greatest power to elders who, in their lifetimes, ascend to posts with increasing prestige and, second, it politically sanctions the practice of civic and religious traditions about which elders have greatest historical perspective.[10]

While Oaxaca is so culturally vibrant because of its myriad communities, the state is also known as a place of significant economic hardship. In 2014, during the time of this study, Oaxaca was one of the poorest states in Mexico (second to Chiapas), with more than 66 percent of the state's population living in poverty and 28 percent meeting criteria for extreme poverty (CONEVAL, 2016). Systemic and social stigma against indigenous people that arose through post-independence and revolutionary ideology help begin to contextualize Oaxaca's poverty, although it is an oversimplification to simply trace the origin of one phenomenon as the consequence of the other.[11] Further, Mexico's neoliberal policies that were implemented during the 1980s have also exasperated these social disparities (Haber, Klein, Maurer, & Middlebrook, 2008, pp. 66–77). With the goal to create more-fluid economic exchange across borders, to privatize and deregulate industries, and to reduce government spending in social programs, Mexico's economic role has grown in the global sphere—but at a cost to the regions that did not (or could not) join. Across Mexico, indigenous communities

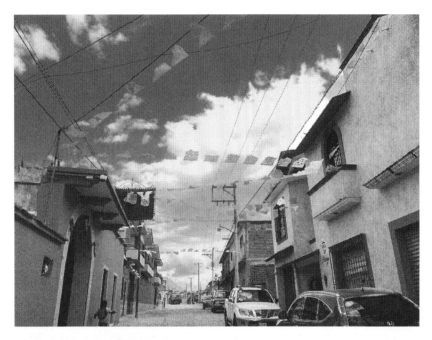

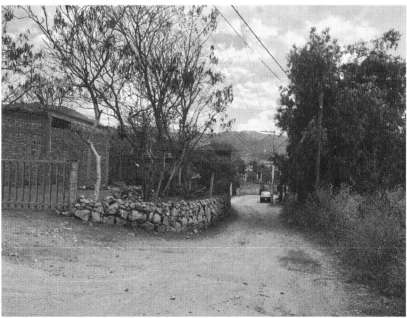

FIGS. i.1a & i.1b. Commercial and rural roads in Teotitlán. *Photographs by the author.*

like Teotitlán experienced these neoliberal trends as a larger campaign to jettison local traditions (Stephen, 2013). Joining the global economy meant adopting national and international (nonindigenous) languages, adhering to foreign legal customs, migrating, and more generally replacing forms of life once centered on communal solidarity and subsistence farming for those premised on social independence and capital gain.[12] These macro-level changes have had a significant impact on local life. For example, upon countless occasions during my research, I was told that life has changed in Teotitlán primarily because people are now preoccupied about finances. Indeed, although the far majority of homes are on family property and there is no demand to pay rent in Teotitlán, households still have to pay *impuesto predial* (property taxes), money for food, and other basic expenditures such that I encountered a general concern about finances. "Before, the corn grew easily and you could always count on having a roof over your head," one informant told me. "Now, that's just not enough—people are always worried about making enough money to survive."

Yet in 2014, when I first arrived in Teotitlán, I was struck by how the community differed from its rural neighbors. In one way, Teotitlán had an active economy and an abundance of signs of relative financial success. From my very first visit I noticed the presence of automobiles (some with U.S.-issued license plates), "smart" mobile phones, and other trending technologies. Part of Teotitlán's success stems from its fortunate geographic positioning. In contrast to the difficult roads that isolate many of Oaxaca's communities, the highway to Teotitlán is a straight, twenty-mile shot from Oaxaca City in the eastern foothills of the Y-shaped *Valles Centrales* (Central Valleys). Here the land is gentle, expansive, and navigable, contrasting with the state's notorious surroundings. This renders easy access to and from Oaxaca City, the region's largest economic hub and representative image of capitalist, "modern" life. Indeed, Teotitlán's physical location and economic positioning place it at the symbolic intersection between two idealized lifestyles: "traditional" life indexed to Teotiteco heritage that draws upon notions of local custom and communal solidarity, and "modern" life indexed to Oaxaca City, Mexico City, California, and other locations where global capitalism and social independence are embraced.

Teotitlán has occupied this intersection in important ways and, in order to appreciate what is at stake in local life, one must attend to the social dynamics that situate it. In part, this concerns Teotitecos' adaptation to the tourist market and related folkloric nationalism as the community positions itself as traditional, indigenous weavers.[13] To be sure, and in comparison to the majority of research on Teotitlán, this book is not about weaving or the larger textile industry. Yet it would be impossible to study Teotitlán without attending to this economic and social mainstay, especially given the way it so dominantly shadowed in the background for the entirety of my fieldwork. Across Oaxaca and the global textile industry, Teotitlán has gained fame for its tapetes, textiles that are often touted as genuine products of Zapotec culture. Many products incorporate motifs from nearby ancient ruins and are celebrated as emblems of Mexico's indigenous history.[14] The sale of tapetes comprises such a large portion of the local economy that it is perhaps an understatement to claim that weaving defines Teotitlán. Undoubtedly, it is Oaxacans' first association to the community and a major self-embraced community characteristic. An overwhelming majority of individuals and households I would come to encounter were involved in the weaving process, and some participants in this study even wove while being interviewed. Yet as Lynn Stephen (2005) and W. Warner Wood (2008) have noted in their own illuminating studies on the community, Teotitlán's involvement in the textile industry complicates how locals create notions of identity: to outside tourists, Teotitecos project a broad, cohesive image of Zapotec ethnicity and themselves as originators of Oaxacan weaving, while among themselves, Teotitecos maintain a narrower sense of identity in a similar way to neighboring communities, centered on local rites and communal practices that differentiate them from neighbors.[15]

While this contributes to an important, nuanced perspective of local identity, the impact of regional poverty and related migration patterns are perhaps equally vital to appreciate local life and what is at stake in it. Yes, Teotitlán has been relatively successful in capitalizing on Oaxacan tourism and textile demands. Stephen (2005) traces how some Teotitecos leveraged economic circumstances (such as the economic crisis during the 1980s that resulted in a "thinning" of middlemen) that enabled locals to become merchants and comparatively wealthy. Wood (2008) discusses how Teotitecos are simultaneously positioned within a local economy, selling textiles at home, and the larger capitalist system that enables locals to engage with the global economy.

These economic shifts have led to relative economic success. But the community is still not exempt from regional poverty and, like many of its Oaxacan neighbors, Teotitecos have migrated in response to it (J. Cohen, 2004; Holmes, 2013; Stephen, 2007).[16] The community continues to receive federal subsidies, and during the time of my research it was designated a poor pueblo by national standards: 82 percent of residents met federal criteria for poverty, and 29 percent lived in extreme poverty (SEDESOL, 2014). This is why, apart from money made

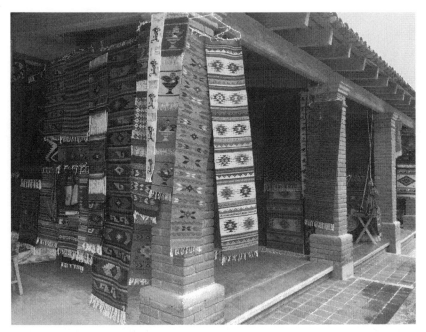

FIG. i.2. Rugs at Teotitlán's tourist market. *Photograph by the author.*

through textile sales in Oaxaca, a significant amount of Teotitlán's economy derives from remittances sent by migrants, and it is estimated that this makes up 17 percent of the state's GDP, sending 1.3 billion dollars per year to local Oaxacan communities (Stephen, 2007, p. 10; Worthen, 2012, p. 6).

For the past 100 years, Oaxacans have migrated to Oaxaca City, Mexico City, and across the U.S.–Mexico border.[17] This significantly impacts what is at stake in the community and further leads to important redefinitions of what local identity means. In the United States, to look at one side of the dynamic, migrants have established "mini" Teotiteco communities where they maintain community-specific customs, speak Zapotec, and continue to identify with the locality of Teotitlán.[18] Among other cities in other U.S. states, in California these communities are based in locations such as Santa Ana, Oxnard, and, to my surprise, Moorpark, which is just a ten-minute drive from my own hometown. Indeed, one of my most extraordinary initial experiences in Teotitlán was the ease with which I was able to converse about my own background. When I lived in Pittsburgh, Pennsylvania, where I attended graduate school, I could only vaguely state that I grew up in a town "north of Los Angeles." But in Teotitlán

I was amazed to be able to talk about specific hometown streets, shopping complexes, and other cultural markers of my youth. In this way, but in contrast to Murphy and Stepick (1991), who claim that Oaxacan migrants jettison traditional customs (p. 129), Teotitlán's migrant communities have become extensions for local Teotiteco practice. They constitute what Michael Kearney (1995) calls "Oaxacalifornia," a type of transnationalized space where Oaxacan migrants physically live abroad but continue to uphold "local" forms of identity (see also Cruz-Manjarrez, 2013). As Stephen (2007) has noted in her important work on "transborder lives," this shifts what local identity means: no longer constituted by the physical borders of Teotitlán, identity is now transnationally stretched and defined by common history, remembrance, and practice of local customs of the community—regardless of where one is physically located.

And conversely, for individuals who remain in Oaxaca, while studies often focus on migrant-sending communities as being the site of significant social hardship, Teotitlán was also not the ghost town described of other Oaxacan settings (for example, Worthen, 2012).[19] The active economy, apparent municipal functioning, and vibrant regularity of *fiestas* testified that Teotitlán was affected but certainly not depleted by migration. This is what makes Teotitlán so interesting to study. Migrants who left often returned, and also continued to make their presence felt from afar. They sent remittances, clothing, and kept in touch over the phone and Internet. Once, on a return flight to Oaxaca from California, I met a Teotiteco who was visiting Teotitlán for three days to attend the confirmation of a godchild. Indeed, the resounding presence of California *within* Teotitlán was salient in nearly every local interaction I'd had. This is even reflected in the Zapotec word for the United States—*Stub Laad*—which translates to mean "the other side," gesturing toward the perceived normality of crossing the international border, and how this process is experienced as being within reach from whatever side one is located.[20]

And yet, for those who remain, migration has a significant impact on everyday life regarding how local identity is defined and social cohesion is maintained. In Teotitlán nearly each household I encountered had a close family member living abroad, and there existed an unspoken community dynamic of the remaining residents coming together to re-form a sense of cohesion. "It does affect me, but it has to be so," said one caregiver of the absences in her family owing to migration. "If they were here they would be helping me. But I'm aware they're not here on a daily basis, and I understand their reason that they're not here." Indeed, there is a strong sense of acceptance of the perceived necessity of those who leave

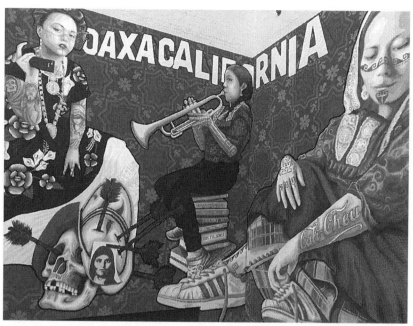

FIG. i.3. *Oaxacalifornia* mural, by the Tlacolulokos. Exhibited at the Los Angeles
Central Library, 2018. Illustrating transborder lifestyles, this mural merges Oaxacan
heritage (represented by traditional attire, *greca* patterns, brass music, and local histories) with Californian influences (represented by modern technology, tattoos, hand
signs, and Euro-American literature). *Photograph by the author. Used by permission of the artists.*

the community to pursue economic ends abroad. Yet this reality creates tension
about local identity and its maintenance. Much like Émile Durkheim (1933/1997)
described of the fragmentation and individualism that societies faced while
becoming more industrialized, in Teotitlán high rates of migration mean that many
households are fragmented, while migrants' return to the community introduces
global influences to local ways of life. Monolingual Zapotec elders stand in
contrast to Spanish-speaking youths, and, in general, locals seemed concerned
to maintain familial and communal solidarity in the face of larger social change.
Ultimately, these social trends mean that one cannot make a firm distinction
between local and global influences; rather, as writers like W. Warner Wood
(2000, 2008) argue, we must appreciate how the global is present within the local
(see also Marcus, 1995; Ruiz Balzola, 2014; Stephen, 2007). This is vital toward
understanding the complexity of social life in Teotitlán—the way that Oaxaca is

said to be tied in knots. Teotitecos maintain a hyperlocal sense of identity while being so directly situated in the broader global world. For those abroad, these social dynamics stretch citizenship to transcend the physical parameters of the community while, for those remaining, they create a felt imperative to maintain local identity and social cohesion in the context of broader social change.

This entire scene—the way local identity is constituted within broader global influence and social change—also comes to directly situate the nature of caregiving itself. Whereas household units were once expected to support and care for dependent elders, now those individual family members who physically remain present are assigned that task. And, whereas the community justifies caring for elders as a matter of social cohesion and local tradition, engagement with the broader global economy also creates tension through an alternative lifestyle based on social independence and capital gain. In sum, how Teotitecos navigate these dynamics, and come to redefine what social cohesion looks like, concretely matters to understand the nature of care on a local level.

A GLOBAL PERSPECTIVE ON CULTURE AND TRADITION

The complexity of Oaxacan social life also puts into focus the basic meaning of local culture and tradition. Teotitecos routinely speak of the fact that they are a traditional community and there is a felt imperative to maintain this claim. Notions of local tradition capture the pulse of social life in Teotitlán, but there is no single practice, value, or outlook that defines what tradition concretely embodies. Language differences, religious and civic customs, and other practices are employed to distinguish Teotitlán from neighboring communities, but the larger gestalt that tradition represents exceeds the sum of its parts. Tradition in Teotitlán is representative of a particular lifestyle as a whole, and concerns about tradition involve questions about its maintenance and regeneration in the context of broader social change.

The presence of new technologies, the absence associated with individuals who have migrated, and related structural and social shifts all demonstrate that Teotitlán is experiencing significant cultural change—but none of this suggests that Teotitlán is becoming any less Teotiteco. As James Clifford (1986) writes, " 'culture' is always relational" (p. 15, with original and deliberate scare quotes on "culture" to avoid implying it is a static object).[21] This is a similar point made by W. Warner Wood (2008) in his own study of Teotitlán when he argues that the Zapotec culture that is celebrated as being definitive of Teotiteco textiles is not something that has survived global forces, but is rather a product of those forces.

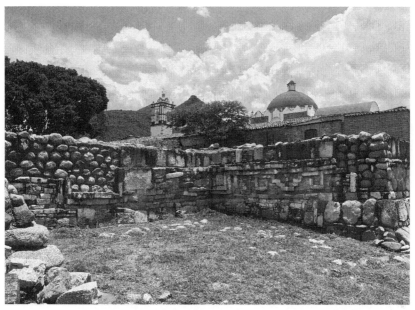

FIG. i.4. Zapotec temple ruins in Teotitlán, over which the Catholic church now stands (in the background). Also in the background is the mountain from which Teotitlán derives its name, *Xigie*, which translates to mean "enchanted" and "below the stones." This location is known locally as the site where the snake god *Quetzalcoatl* appeared and prophesied to the then-nomadic people of Oaxaca that they should settle and give birth to the Zapotec civilization. *Photograph by the author.*

This includes how "non-Zapotec" influences like Navajo designs and colors have been incorporated into Teotiteco textiles. Wood turns to anthropologist Richard Wilk (2006), whom he credits with this perspective. Wilk asks:

> Does local culture persist *despite* globalization, like a nail that will not be hammered down? . . . Or could it be that there is something about globalization itself that produces local culture? . . . We have been so convinced that colonization and globalization are forces of homogenization and the domination of local cultures by modernizing and globalizing Euro-American culture that it takes a real effort to switch gears and consider this possibility. (p. 10)

In this way, changes to the community do not contradict the way Teotitecos purport to be traditional; rather, they help justify tradition itself.

In this book I take "tradition"—and notions about why caring for elders is an instance of tradition—not as a timeless and anchored construct that remains constant, but rather as a set of repeated practices passed across generations that constantly evolves in response to surrounding circumstances. For example, whereas historically Teotitecos made a short pilgrimage to the rock believed to be the site where the snake-god *Quetzalcoatl* prophesized the birth of Zapotec civilization, today individuals travel to the same place as Catholics to celebrate the Day of the Holy Cross.[22] And, in reference to the pre-Hispanic belief that deceased ancestors return to safeguard the community, Teotitecos now celebrate *Dia de Los Muertos* within a Catholic framework through All Saints' Day. In so many ways, cultural syncretism is not the exception but the norm, and traditions do not become extinct but are adapted to fit within the changing social landscape. All this to say that tradition does not oppose but is constituted within modernity, and is best understood as a set of practices that arises and regenerates in the context of broader social change (see Fabian, 2014; Graburn, 2001; Horner, 1990).[23]

Although Teotitecos themselves understand social life in terms of a binary between tradition and modernity, these temporal idioms implicitly reference ideas about progress and backwardness. And this, in turn, is based on larger political campaigns that define progress via engagement with capitalism and related forms of industrial life (Pigg, 1996). This is also why any analysis of modernity is problematic; whenever it is mentioned, one inherently posits something it is not—the premodern, traditional, or archaic—thereby producing the category differences that define its meaning (Latour, 1993; see also Clifford & Marcus, 1986). Yet while I am aware of the problematic dichotomy between tradition and modernity, I employ both terms because they are so commonly used in everyday Teotiteco life, and also because they situate the topic of this investigation. As I come to show, Alzheimer's disease and other forms of age-related forgetfulness are understood as modern conditions, associated with the stresses seen to result from engaging with capitalistic, nontraditional lifestyles. And concomitantly, family caregiving is understood as a practice that upholds traditional values centered on family, social cohesion, and respect for elders in the context of broader cultural change. These social categories have local significance, yet my use of them does not suggest that life in Teotitlán is somehow categorically different than some earlier period in time, or that there are somehow distinct traditional and modern modes of being. I do not take modernity to be a totalizing, discrete way of life that is standard across time and place, and neither do I purport to claim that Teotitlán is experiencing a "transition" to modernity. Rather, I see modernity and tradition as concomitant perspectives of the same contemporary experience. Yes, life is qualitatively different than it was in the past, but much to Wilk's point, what is taken to be "traditional" is inextricably constituted within the features of contemporary life.

DEMENTIA CAREGIVING AS SOCIAL REGENERATION

Caregiving for dementia is a primary analytic to observe how cultural practices and social relations regenerate in the context of broader social change. In Teotitlán, elders are representative of social cohesion in three senses: as possessing knowledge of local tradition; as living anchors to the historical past; and as recipients of care that itself embodies the act of people coming together. This is why age-related forgetfulness provides a specifically helpful vista for studying social cohesion. Elders who face difficulty remembering have more reason to be cared for, but their forgetfulness also begets uncertainty about how they can be heralded as local authorities who have command over social rites. And conversely for caregivers, the custom of drawing upon younger generations to care for elders is put in question as greater numbers migrate and households are fragmented. Again, the point is not to suggest that these tensions undermine caregiving or broader Teotiteco culture; rather, the questions they raise help illustrate how both are (re)constituted within and responsive to broader social changes.

Contemporary work on the anthropology of care has centered on this exact point. In contrast to previous trends that viewed caregiving as a practice of social reproduction, scholars have recently revised this perspective to take account of the dynamic and fluid social factors that constantly evolve and mutually constitute it. Earlier research viewed caregiving as an act of social *reproduction* and thus understood care as an interpersonal resource that maintains biological and social life (Baxter & Almagor, 1978; Goody, 1976). People care for others to help others survive. While there is obvious truth in this perspective, social reproductive perspectives are based on a functionalist framework that assumes a constancy in social systems; here, care is seen as something that reproduces and sustains life across generations, not as something that is inherently responsive to dynamic changes within them.[24] That is why scholars like Cole and Durham (2015), Kristin Yarris (2017), and others argue that viewing care as a social reproductive practice is problematic; it does not take into account how caregiving itself is adaptive and redefined within broader contexts. Hence, instead of viewing caregiving as a practice of reproduction, they suggest it is better understood as a practice of *regeneration*, accounting for social change by emphasizing the "mutually constitutive interplay between intergenerational relations and wider historical and social processes" (Cole & Durham, 2015, p. 17).

Appreciating caregiving as a regenerative practice highlights how it involves new forms of relating to family members and the larger community. This concerns what I call the segre-social dynamics of caregiving for forgetful elders in Teotitlán, an admittedly clumsy term that attempts to capture how caregivers are simultaneously drawn into new familial relations centered on dementia but, in so doing, risk becoming misunderstood by and segregated from the larger community. In part, this term draws on the verb *to segregate* (from Latin *segregare*, "to set apart, lay aside; isolate; divide," literally "separate from the flock"). At the same time, the term also addresses how caregiving generates new forms of social life, new ways for family members to come together under the provision of care. To the latter point, this term gestures to the rich line of anthropological research on "biosociality," an analytical frame that attends to the way biological conditions like Alzheimer's disease generate new forms of social life such as the formation Alzheimer's support groups, novel encounters with medical professionals, and other forms of social behavior centered on this condition (Lock, 2007; Rabinow, 1996; Rose, 2007). Further, to engage with more recent studies in Oaxaca, this term is also situated within Whitney Duncan's (2018) research on the emergence of a "psy-sociality" generated by foreign concepts in mental health that lead to novel ways for individuals to come together to understand and process psychological conflict. In addition to these social forms, the segre-social dynamics of this book capture the paradoxical experience of Teotitecos' desire for sociofamilial cohesion while recognizing that the maintenance of one in the home risks the foreclosure of the other in the community. Family members choose to care for elders as an instance of upholding local values about respect for elders, as a means of maintaining social cohesion, but in so doing, the larger community can hold them responsible for elders' decline. As I will come to show, caregivers are blamed owing to local understandings about age-related forgetfulness as a modern (nontraditional) condition that is held to not exist in Teotitlán.

This is part of a larger perspective of how caregiving reveals and regenerates key local values inherent to the cohesion of the community. In this book I draw upon literature on the anthropology of care to explore how caregivers at once justify their commitment to forgetful elders through appealing to local values while, in so doing, expose tensions inherent to maintaining those values in contemporary life. Researchers have variously analyzed caregiving as an ethical practice that recuperates social relations in the context of shrinkage to state-sponsored social programs (Garcia, 2010; Han, 2012), a critical response to the prioritization of "hypercognitive" Western values over relational and emotive ones (Kitwood, 1997; Post, 2000), an adaptive strategy to maintain social cohesion in the context of transnational migration (Leinaweaver, 2010; Parreñas, 2005; Yarris, 2017), and a practice that generates new forms of morality and subjectivity in the context of social change (Buch, 2013). Each of these analytical frames contains an underlying assumption about caregiving as a practical response to ethical issues inherent in a dynamically shifting social world. That is why anthropologists like Arthur Kleinman (2008) have gone so far as to generalize that "caregiving is a foundational component of moral experience . . . [that is best understood as] an existential quality of what it is to be a human being" (p. 23). It is through humanely responding to another person in times of need that we not only sustain another's biological life, but also manifest the qualities that define us as social beings dependent on care from others. It is these latter qualities that capture how and why caregiving is meaningful, and what is perceived to be at stake for caregivers in their daily lives.

This book accounts for how caregiving embodies a human ethic to attend to others in need. At the same time, it remains anchored in a cultural anthropology that is sensitive to the way ethical sensibilities are specifically constituted within—and dynamically regenerated in response to—broader circumstances in Teotitlán's social landscape. This further builds on what Mol, Moser, and Pols (2010) have aptly labeled the "ethics of care," an overarching approach to study caregiving not as generating prescriptive answers about what leads to a good life, but rather exploring how notions about the good are negotiated in everyday caregiving practice. In their words, "The good is not something to pass a judgment on . . . but something to *do*, in practice, as care goes on" (p. 13). To make sense of how the good is performed in caregiving, this book focuses on the phenomenology of ethical injunctions to maintain values about social cohesion *qua* caregiving and, in so doing, studies how social relations are redefined in the process.

Woven throughout this book's presentation of caregiving voices is analysis regarding how values are pragmatically defined and concretely practiced. In Teotitlán, notions of what makes life good and assessments about whether individuals are measuring up to this standard are embedded within larger social issues about the importance of maintaining local identity and social cohesion. These issues point to how social relations like caregiving are not merely a process of upholding values about respect for elders and local tradition, but also involve their regeneration by taking into account and responding to broader social dynamics.

EPISTEMOLOGICAL CONSIDERATIONS

In part, this approach to studying caregiving draws on social constructionism, a theoretical perspective that defines the majority of anthropological research and attends to cultural differences in the way phenomena like illnesses, social relations, and moral commitments are constructed within (or, constitutive of) specific social worlds.[25] Social constructionism helps account for how such phenomena might mean something different across time and place, but it does not go further to appreciate how these differences are important to study and serve local functions in their own right. It is not enough to merely observe that illness experience varies across time and place; to genuinely appreciate and sensitively attend to these differences, we must also inquire what function they locally serve and how they respond to the values at stake in everyday life. As a clinician, this is to me an especially important issue because, however much one might attend to the way different cultures have varying experiences of illness, we are still liable to assume that some understandings are more valid than others and thus overlook appreciation for why difference matters. This latter concern is especially important in mental health, where clinicians tend to translate and reduce different expressions of illness into a framework (biomedical, cognitive, psychoanalytic, and so forth) that we prefer to operate within, as an instance of chemical imbalance, inaccurate thinking, repression, and so forth. And further, we tend to translate between illness categories themselves: *susto* (fright, in Latin American cultures) is taken as a symptom of depression, *khyâl* attacks (wind attacks, among Cambodians) are understood as expressions of anxiety, and so on. In being reframed, experiences of illness are emptied of their local meanings, including the specifics of what is distressing about illness and why individuals are motivated to seek help in the first place (see Abramowitz, 2010; Merry, 2006).

This is not only a problem among mental health workers, but also for the majority of researchers who attempt to study culture while implicitly maintaining that there exists a realm of scientific knowledge that transcends it. There is an epistemological fissure between scientific knowledge and cultural competence, leading anthropologist Byron Good (1994) to rather provokingly write that even the study of " 'Medical anthropology' is a kind of oxymoron" (p. 176). Good's point is that while anthropologists approach the topics of their research as being constituted within specific social settings, many also paradoxically use the term "medical" to refer to an underlying, objective realm of science that cuts across these social parameters.[26] Such tendencies reveal an "underlying epistemological ambivalence" that situates medical anthropology (Good, 1994, p. 28) and, for the same reason, an ambivalence among clinicians as well. When, for example, one knows about Alzheimer's disease as a neurological disorder that involves underlying plaques and tangles, as a condition involving genetic susceptibility for early-onset cases, and an illness whose prevalence rates generally manifest the same globally, it is difficult to encounter contrary perspectives and think they are, in fact, not erroneous. It is difficult to assume an alternative to the perspective that the important knowledge gained from empirical science reflects the world's natural order and that scientific advancements about illness are true across time and place.

To be sure, there *is* something objective about science—and I would be foolish to argue otherwise. And yet, in maintaining this stance, we fail to appreciate what Joel Robbins (2013) terms the "cultural point" in anthropology and, for that matter, the point in all efforts that aim for cultural competence. The point is that cultural differences run deep and constitute fundamental aspects of human experience, including health and illness. It concretely matters that in Teotitlán, Alzheimer's and age-related forgetfulness not only have an underlying neurological truth, but a cultural one as well. This is a truth that positions the threat of forgetfulness as a larger concern about social change, a truth that informs the various meanings, everyday experiences, and social relationships into a distinct reality about forgetfulness that must be attended to in itself. Overlooking this fact omits much of what forgetfulness means and the specific ways it is distressing. Yet to appreciate such truths in their own light involves a radical shift in how cultural knowledge is perceived: away from viewing knowledge as a type of "mirror of nature" that remains constant and valid across cultural settings, and toward appreciating "knowledge as a matter of conversation and of social practice" that varies and is relative to time and place (Rorty, 1979, p. 171). Anthropologists appear correct in suggesting that this epistemological shift is necessary in order to genuinely approach and appreciate how various cultures might hold alternative views about illness.

As an effort toward the latter, this book considers how the local meaning of age-related forgetfulness represents a truth in its own right and serves functions specific to the Teotiteco community. To accomplish this, this book engages with pragmatism, a philosophical cousin to social constructionism, known for challenging the assumption that truth is objective and constant, transcendent and universal—a dominant set of assumptions in much of philosophy since Plato—and instead embracing an alternative epistemology that focuses on how various *truths* are useful in a given time and place. Pragmatists like William James (1907/2000), John Dewey (1929/1998), Charles Pierce (1905), and more recent scholars hold that truth is not an abstract, inherent property of ideas, but rather a creative process wherein an idea is placed in relation to others held to be true.[27] As James (1907/2000) observed, "The truth of an idea is not a stagnant property inherent in it. Truth happens to an idea. It *becomes* true, is made true by events" (p. 88).

In this book, pragmatism proves an important analytic frame to situate a view of dementia that does not somehow purport to attend to local meanings while implicitly assuming that some forms of knowledge are more accurate than others. Rather, it takes into account how local truths, strategies, and experiences of dementia serve purposes specific to the Teotiteco community. With a pragmatic lens we not only appreciate how the experience of dementia is passively construct*ed* within a given social world (a perspective offered from the social constructionists), but also how it is functionally construct*ive* of the world people want to furnish. To again borrow from James (1907/2000), pragmatism attends to the "practical cash value" of what dementia means locally, and how this truth makes a concrete difference in everyday life (p. 28).

This approach—call it cultural pragmatism—offers a way to "bracket" what has become a natural assumption among clinicians to understand illness via scientific parameters, and to simultaneously attend to illness in the context of those who experience it.[28] Cultural pragmatism at once refers to the everyday pragmatic sensibility clinicians need while working with different populations— to be pragmatically useful and to adapt to the needs of different individuals—but it also refers to an epistemological perspective that allows clinicians to appreciate how and why different truths can be valid. Further, in using this term, I deliberately invoke the idea of bracketing from the phenomenological tradition, which acknowledges the presence of a commonsensical attitude about there being an underlying objective reality, but encourages this attitude to be put aside to study human experience in its own light (Husserl, 1913/1963).[29] While phenomenologists had their own agenda, the idea of bracketing is useful toward appreciating how truth can simultaneously refer to objective scientific truth *and*, from the pragmatist's perspective, the truth of immediate experience of illness that differs across time and place. This latter form of truth is one that attends to contingency, as well as social function.

Bracketing seems especially important today in a world of "alternative facts," "fake news," and other allegations that question basic instances of common knowledge. My approach in this book is not to provide more ammunition for what I see as a dangerous social trend—and not to use social constructionism, pragmatism, or issues pertaining to culture as a means to undermine scientific objectivity. Rather, my goal is to begin to develop an epistemology that attends to culture as constituting a truth in itself—one that stands on the same epistemological footing as scientific ones. This is an epistemology that appreciates how various truths function in the service of social cohesion and, again, not one that uses those truths to undermine scientific knowledge. As Bruno Latour (2004) writes, the whole point of this approach is not to somehow get away from facts, but rather to come closer to them. In the case of this book, the facts we come closer to concern facts about human experience, what illness means in context, and how people come together in its presence. In Latour's words, "The critic is not the one who debunks, but the one who assembles . . . not the one who lifts the rug from under the feet of the naïve believers, but the one who offers the participants arenas in which to gather" (p. 246). In this approach, researchers and clinicians not only witness how other people assemble together through their own specific truths, but also come closer to the subjects they study and treat through the act of respectful listening.

In general, bracketing the natural attitude about scientific naturalism provides a view of illness that is not only attentive to its cultural variants, but also a way to appreciate how those variants shape basic experience about illness. Cultural pragmatism provides a way to attend to differences across cultures and appreciate how those differences function to bring people together. And, equally important, engaging with pragmatism is helpful to capture the heart of the voices presented in this book—as I will come to show, these are caregivers who were concerned not to strictly follow one medical strategy over another, but individuals who dynamically adopted multiple (and at times contradictory) strategies to deliver the best intended and most effective care to loved ones in the context of broader social change.

METHODS: LOCAL CHALLENGES
AND STRATEGIC RESPONSES

From the very beginning of fieldwork, this project faced numerous challenges. I wanted to gain information about the local experience of caregiving for elders living with dementia, but I quickly realized this was tantamount to inquiring about the intimate details of strangers' lives. And, while I had arrived to Oaxaca intent on asking about Alzheimer's and related forms of dementia, most people told me that it simply did not exist. In so many ways, access proved a continuous hurdle that marked the entirety of my research experience. Yet instead of forcing the setting of my research into something it was not, I embraced the obstacles I encountered and, in so doing, transformed them into advantageous points of entry. I well recognize that a "methods" section has fallen out of fashion in contemporary texts, but in what follows I outline methods used because they further contextualize the scene of this research and how I began to orient myself to it.

To start, Teotitlán's pride in distinguishing itself from neighboring communities meant that internal cohesion was maintained through exclusion of those outside. And, precisely because I was not from Teotitlán, Oaxaca, or Mexico, people viewed me with a considerable lack of *confianza* (confidence, trust).[30] This became a major obstacle throughout my research because, unlike how I was accustomed to building trust with new acquaintances in the United States through mutual interest in respective differences, the lack of confianza I faced in Teotitlán was premised precisely on who and what I was not.[31] This was a reality I encountered again and again. As one family whom I had tried to speak with for months told me, "People need time, they need confianza."

As if this did not pose enough of a hurdle, when I spoke to people about my interest in studying dementia and Alzheimer's disease in particular, nearly every individual stated that they had either never heard of Alzheimer's or that it simply did not exist in Teotitlán. This was something Alex told me upon first meeting him, as well as other residents, community leaders, and allopathic and traditional health providers. As I will elaborate in chapter 2, I came to realize that Alzheimer's was understood as a modern condition that occurred in response to the stresses associated with nontraditional ways of living. Individuals wanted to believe Alzheimer's did not exist and, of those who knew otherwise, there was strong reluctance to speak about it.

Initially, I sought Alex's help because the literature I had read in preparation of research had alerted me that, although a growing number of younger individuals speak Spanish, the majority of social life is carried out in Zapotec, and that most elders experienced difficulty sustaining deep conversation in Spanish. I did not want to limit whom I could interview, and I also anticipated meeting with spouses of elders (whom I anticipated would likely be monolingual). Yet I soon came to realize that Alex was more than a hired translator: he was a critical

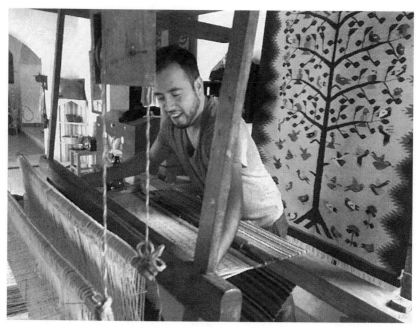

FIG. i.5. Alex weaving. *Photograph by the author.*

figure to facilitate the type of "border crossing" I sought in meeting with locals and to understand the nuanced dimensions of their lived experience (Temple & Edwards, 2008).

Indeed, although it may be unconventional to so centrally feature Alex's involvement, I am deliberately emphasizing his role as a matter of justice and accuracy. As Russ Walsh (2003) notes, the type of qualitative research I aimed to conduct has a significant tradition of embracing reflexivity that "turns back upon or takes account of" the research process. That is why, included in my study of caregivers and the broader Teotiteco community, I also studied Alex and his participation in the project. This approach responds to Catherine Riessman's (2002) challenge to "do justice" in research by featuring more than one voice. While Riessman is concerned to involve her participants in writing research results, I take a slightly different approach by framing "my" methods as an interpersonal endeavor that could not have been achieved independently. Here, justice involves acknowledging that this project would not have been possible without Alex's commitment to it.[32]

The way in which Alex took this investigation as his own increasingly fostered greater trust among his neighbors. Strangers whom I would later come to meet said that they knew of me as that *gringo* associated with Alex. They sensed that because Alex was willing to place his trust in me, others could as well. And, in response to the disconcerting reality that every local professed that Alzheimer's did not exist, Alex and I strategized to give up inquiring about Alzheimer's disease and dementia nominally, and instead look for symptoms of forgetfulness among elders. The Zapotec word *rienlá'az* (to forget) became our catchword.[33] This made sense given the stigma that surrounded dementia and allowed me to present my interests with less cause for alarm.[34]

In the course of these efforts, I leveraged my partnership with Alex to develop a collaborative interviewing strategy that transformed the initial obstacles I faced into strategic points of entry. Responding to the way in which confianza and Zapotec were prioritized in ordinary conversations, Alex and I identified the most salient questions of my research interests in order for *him* to carry out discussions with households in Zapotec. We drew on techniques from focus group interviewing and tailored our approach to leverage his linguistic advantage to maximize group discussions and minimize my participation as researcher (Carey & Smith, 1994; Kidd & Parshall, 2000; Krueger, 2009).[35] Having Alex conduct interviews with households not only facilitated access to a community that initially viewed me with susipicion, but also fostered collection of data that was more ecologically valid given that in Oaxaca it is the household—not the individual—that constitutes the primary social unit (J. Cohen, 2004; Murphy & Stepick, 1991; Norget, 2006).[36]

After each interview, we met to translate and transcribe audio recordings, typically before moving on to the next. This provided another opportunity to reflect on how to improve our technique. We met at Alex's home or mine, in front of two computers—one for him to control the audio, and another for me to transcribe. This process was arduous and sometimes amounted to more than ten hours spent transcribing for every one hour of recording. Yet it was significantly informative. Often, Alex encountered a word or concept that had no equivalent translation. He either tried to find a phrase using a combination of Spanish and English words or, more often, paused to explain local concepts that were too difficult to capture in a single phrase. For example, one participant used the Zapotec word *anim*, which roughly translates to "soul." Alex explained that this translation is only approximate because it is used specifically to describe the soul of the deceased. (The Zapotec word *garlieng* is used to describe the soul of a living person.) Transcribing not only gave me a chance to unpack what occurred during interviews—to witness the way caregiving was discussed by family members and Alex—but it also provided an opportunity to further question a member of the community about the broader significance of the data we were gathering.

Through the course of a year of fieldwork partnering with Alex and other activities pertinent to this study, in Teotitlán we interviewed twenty-two family caregivers for elders living with dementia across nine households (comprising more than fifteen hours of recorded interviews conducted in Zapotec). All interview data were subsequently analyzed and, throughout writing up findings, I continued to reread interview transcripts to ensure that presentation of data was harmonious with the overall interview.[37] These local perspectives were supplemented by other interviews with community doctors, *curanderas* (traditional healers), psychologists, state-employed individuals who work with elders, and other relationships made in the course of this study. I took detailed field notes throughout and also attended *pláticas*, fiestas and public celebrations, and shared countless encounters with other locals.[38] Lastly, I formally studied the Zapotec language (the dialect spoken in Teotitlán) to better understand local customs and continue developing access to the community.[39]

I well recognize that many anthropologists might take objection to my approach. It is commonly expected that investigators fluently speak the language of those whom they study to reduce interpersonal distance. Yet having Alex spark conversation among household members fostered rich data—not between participants and me, but more importantly among participants as they talked among themselves.[40] Having Alex available to create a space for conversation—and subsequently having access to him to explain subtle differences (as during the transcription process)—unquestionably gave rise to more intimate data than if I had conducted interviews myself in Zapotec. The fact that Teotitecos differentiated themselves not only from Spanish speakers but also from other Zapotec-speaking neighboring communities provided a constant reminder of the importance of studying *local* dialogue among locals themselves. This goal could not have been achieved by my initiative alone.

As I will illustrate throughout the course of the book, the collaborative approach I developed with Alex helped foster significant information on the specific ways caregivers experience their lives. But it also came to embody a relevant social response to the distress I came to notice within the community. As I began to appreciate, Alex was carrying out conversations with caregivers about their experience—a type of lifestyle he had believed did not exist. And

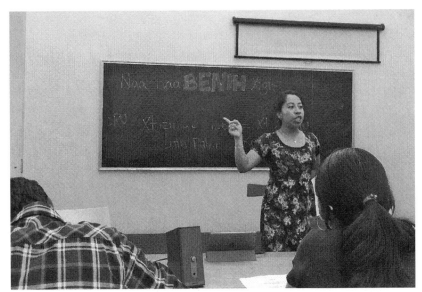

FIG. i.6. Janet Chávez Santiago teaching a Zapotec language class. On the black-
board Janet instructs students how to say *Naa naa benib Xigue,* which translates to
mean, "I am from Teotitlán." *Photograph by the author.*

conversely, caregivers were making known their experience to a representative
of the community who had once been blind to their realities. In this unique
setting, I was able to witness the negotiation of the meaning of caregiving—
not only among family members as they conversed with each other, but also
among families and a citizen of the broader community. In this way, Alex not
only provided access to this unique ethnographic scene, but also enacted what
anthropologists and other qualitative researchers have sought in calling for a
more "engaged" and "activist" style of inquiry.[41] Alex's involvement in recruiting
participants, his learning of the suffering of neighbors' lives, and his conviction
to respond to that suffering all point to the way that doing research also entails
making concrete, social change. This is an underlying theme throughout the
book, but will be most explicitly discussed toward its end.

CHAPTER OUTLINE

In the five chapters that follow, I present analysis of what Buch (2015) terms a
"polysemic understanding of care" for age-related dementia in Teotitlán, that
is, an analysis of the varied meanings, experiences, and behaviors involved in

caregiving, and consideration for how these dimensions are constituted within and responsive to surrounding social dynamics. The multiple frames adopted in this book also speak to my unique stance as a researcher. I write here from a dual psychological-anthropological standpoint and engage with both disciplines in attempting to understand what family caregiving for dementia in Oaxaca can teach us about the intimate, lived experience of contemporary Teotiteco life and, by extension, what such intimacy can reveal about the nature of care and culture. As I will illustrate through the course of the book, this stance engenders respective lessons for each discipline—for psychology, highlighting constraints on its tendencies to master information about culture prior to being taught by patients; for anthropology, in addition to contributing to relevant research on caregiving and Oaxaca, fostering a reflexivity that ethnographic inquiry is, in itself, a form of care.

In this introductory chapter, I have presented Teotitlán as the setting of this book and discuss how aging and dementia serve as a prism to appreciate contemporary social issues facing the community. In general, these issues concern how Teotitecos perceive their community to be changing in the context of global influence and how individuals experience concomitant injunctions to maintain local identity and communal values centered on social-familial cohesion. I have reviewed relevant literature on the anthropology of care and discussed how caregiving, in addition to sustaining life in moments of dependency, can be seen as a social practice that regenerates local values and social relations. I have also introduced cultural pragmatism as providing an epistemological framework that attends to cultural dimensions of illness in their own right. Lastly, I discussed methodological obstacles and strategies used to collect data.

Chapter 1 is focused on social issues concerning aging, dementia, and caregiving in Oaxaca. The chapter first introduces caregivers and their households and subsequently reviews how contemporary caregiving in Teotitlán challenges normative gender and domestic roles. Next, the chapter proceeds to discuss what I term "the problem of aging in Teotitlán"—that is, demographic trends that reveal how elders are more prevalent and growing into later decades than ever before, and are thus increasingly placing demands on their families and community to meet growing needs. Lastly, the chapter reviews local representations of dementia, Alzheimer's disease, and related forms of forgetfulness as indexed to broader concerns about social change. I discuss how age-related forgetfulness is subsequently viewed with stigma and how this perception contributes to the segre-social realities that caregivers endure. Throughout these points, I present relevant historical and theoretical perspectives that help contextualize the nature of phenomena of this study.

Chapter 2 focuses on analyzing idioms of distress pertaining to progressive dementia, what would generally be called Alzheimer's disease in other settings. This chapter is divided into two main sections, respectively focused on what behavioral symptoms caregivers notice in dementia, followed by a section devoted to caregivers' etiological understandings of those symptoms. Overall, this chapter demonstrates how caregivers' idioms are constituted within a medically plural setting and, more importantly, function to uphold household cohesion in the context of larger social change. In developing these themes, this chapter also draws on pragmatism to illustrate its relevance toward appreciating of cultural dimensions of illness.

Chapter 3 continues to develop these themes by turning to study how caregivers make choices regarding whom to (not) consult for professional help, and the social impact of their decisions. This chapter explores the perceived benefits of visiting curanderas versus allopathic doctors, and how this choice is situated within a community that is responding to implicit power dynamics inherent in each system of medicine. In so doing, this chapter contextualizes the last chapter by identifying how larger discursive realms of power also shape health-seeking behavior.

Chapter 4 focuses on caregivers' relationships with forgetful elders. This chapter first reviews the common challenges that caregivers experience and how these are viewed in the context of broader social change. Next, the chapter proceeds to discuss how caregiving leads to a novel form of relating to elders and, in so doing, employs the concept of "role reversal" to make sense of this relationship. Lastly, the chapter attends to the concrete, behavioral aspects of caregivers' relationship with elders by observing the way caregivers strategize to respond to the challenges they face.

Chapter 5 expands analysis on caregiving sociality to attend to how caregivers relate to the broader community. In the first part, the chapter studies the local values that caregivers use to justify their caregiving experience, and how appealing to these values is expressive of their attempts to promote family cohesion and engage with the broader community. In the second, the chapter proceeds to explore how caregivers' attempts to uphold these values paradoxically render them on the social periphery. It analyzes how caregivers are forgotten, misunderstood, and subject to gossip by the larger community. This paradoxical dynamic reveals the segre-social dynamics inherent to caregiving and the concomitant social suffering caregivers endure.

The epilogue concludes with a reflection of *La Danza de los Viejos* (The Dance of the Elders), an annual celebration that depicts larger social ambivalence about aging. It considers the collection of findings developed in this study and mobilizes them for broader purposes: for clinicians, how to think about and promote cultural pragmatism; for general readers, how implicit values shape the meaning of aging and age-related illness. These remarks also provide reflection on the nature of caregiving and what lessons might be drawn within anthropology about care in Teotitlán. It concludes with consideration for how this project might carry impact locally, and studies Alex's experience as a lesson on this point.

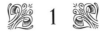

1

The Problem of Aging in Teotitlán

CONTEXTUALIZING CAREGIVERS, ELDERS, AND AGE-RELATED FORGETFULNESS

Pedro is tricky.[1] An elder in his mid-70s, he has begun to forget not only basic things but where he is in the world. He wanders. He tries to escape to the streets when doors are left open, and he hides objects when confined at home. His family is responsible for his care, an experience they say is challenging. "Sometimes I can't take it, taking care of him. Because he gets me so angry," said his youngest son, Sergio. Part of this challenge involves how they make sense of Pedro's behavior. "What I just don't understand is if he uses [his forgetfulness] for his own gain," reflected his eldest son, Manuel. "Because the thing is, he is tricky. He's very tricky. . . . That's why I can't understand if he really forgets or if he's just tricky. So I don't know—it's on him if he's lying to us, or if it's true what's happening to him." Manuel is questioning the basic existence of Alzheimer's. These uncertainties—and the subsequent family tensions they cause—are a dominant occurrence for caregivers in Teotitlán.

Sergio's family home was located on a quiet, paved side street, but he lived within seconds of Teotitlán's main commercial and transportation artery, lined with shops selling colorful *tapetes* and other household provisions. This 30-year-old local was unmarried and well known in Teotitlán for running his family's successful *tortilla* business. After learning about the nature of our project, Sergio

34

warmly smiled and invited us to his home. Inside, the courtyard was paved, with no visible livestock, fruit trees, or weaving looms. The walls consisted of smooth concrete, instead of adobe. There was an overall calm that distinguished private life from public streets. Sergio directed us into the quiet and shaded altar room. It was sparsely decorated, with some wooden chairs lined along the wall. On one side sat a wooden table that served as the family altar. It displayed dated and faded family photographs and a large colorful painting of the crucifixion, alongside fresh-cut flowers and unlit candles.

Sergio invited his 45-year-old brother, Manuel, and Linda, their 65-year-old mother, to join. Compared to his brother, who lived on the same property in his own home with his family and dependent children, Sergio remained at his childhood home, living with his parents. This was a typical arrangement for Teotiteco single adults, who are expected to contribute to family households until having a family of their own. Sergio helped with finances by managing the tortilla business and harvesting *milpa* on communal farmland, but he spent much of his time alongside his brother and mother, directed toward caring for Pedro, their 75-year-old "tricky" and forgetful father. For the past two years, Pedro showed difficulty remembering family member names and often misplaced objects, while accusing others for their disappearance. Pedro also complained of knee pain from having worked in muddy farmlands and displayed signs of visual hallucinations, claiming that snakes were crawling on walls.

But Sergio and his family mainly described how they found other behavioral changes most distressing. On one occasion, Pedro threw a glass bottle at his wife while she was trying to help him bathe, leaving her frightened to approach him for weeks. And just months before my visit, Sergio and his family experienced a more alarming episode during a trip to Tijuana. Pedro wandered away from their relatives' home and went missing. Hours later, after presumably boarding a bus, someone spotted Pedro walking alone in unfamiliar streets. Sergio described his relief that his father was still alive, but in his account of this and other events he also described feeling frustrated and angry:

> I can't tell him not to do something. He'll always do it, anyway. And I can't force him to do something he doesn't want to do. Since he'll just hit me. And he's my dad so of course I can't hit him back, even if he gets me angry. And I personally think that that's a really big problem for me. Because even if he gets me very angry I still try to respect him.

The previous ways Sergio had related to his father stood in contrast to the realities he encountered now. Sergio lived in a community marked by the expectation that parents and elders are respected on account of their age. And, specific to their relationship, Sergio had grown up admiring his father for his household authority and the success he had garnered in establishing the family business. In learning more about the details of this family's experience, it became clear that so much of what they found difficult in caregiving involved the negotiation of social expectations about respect for elders at a time when respect seemed so difficult to locate.

This chapter introduces the details of these social expectations, broadly aiming to trace what old age and related illness mean in a setting marked by social change, and the segre-social dynamics inherent to local caregiving experience. Caregiving represents a new form of social life based on care practices for elders' forgetfulness in a setting that perceives forgetfulness itself as representative of broader, unwanted cultural change. As discussed in the introduction, the segre-social dynamics that interest me are meant to account for this phenomenon. They draw on Paul Rabinow's (1996) pioneering concept of "biosociality," a description where "new group and individual identities and practices" coalesce around public understandings of biology such that everyday life becomes redefined and reorganized by biological conditions themselves (p. 102; see also Nicholas Rose's [2007] concept of "biological citizenship" and Whitney Duncan's [2018] concept of "psy-sociality").[2] For example, as information about Alzheimer's disease circulates in U.S. settings, new forms of social life have subsequently surfaced. The development of caregiver and patient support groups, political lobbying for research funding, education, prevention campaigns, and related activities all foment a different lifestyle with different social relations, essentially "draw[ing] involved families to an [Alzheimer's] society" (Lock, 2007, p. 58). In Oaxaca, caregiving for dementia similarly draws individuals into new social configurations, yet broader understandings of dementia simultaneously can render caregivers misunderstood by and segregated from the larger community. My focus on segre-social dynamics thus accounts for the simultaneous social and segregative dimensions inherent in caregiving. This sociality is representative of novel forms of caregivers' relationships—both with elders and the broader community—while revealing how these relationships are embedded in a community regenerating the meaning of values concerning familial piety, gendered divisions of labor, and broader injunctions to maintain local tradition.

This chapter begins with an introduction to the set of caregiving voices and households that comprise this book, with focus on how caregivers have both affirmed and regenerated normative expectations about the provision of care in the context of migration and related social changes. Following this, I review demographic changes that have altered the Teotiteco social landscape and discuss how these changes lead to novel perceptions of—and challenges associated with—elders' increasing presence in society. Last, I explore local understandings of Alzheimer's disease and more general statements about age-related forgetfulness that are together indexed to concerns about social change, and I begin to consider how these perspectives contribute to the segre-social dynamics caregivers experience. As a whole, this chapter aims to contextualize information important to appreciate subsequent ones. Prior to attending to the cultural pragmatism that is the topic of the remaining chapters of the book, this chapter situates the setting of this study through constructionist theory, addressing how the meaning and experience of basic phenomena like age, illness, and identity are contingent on time and place.

INTRODUCING CAREGIVING HOUSEHOLDS

My decision to interview Sergio with Manuel and Linda is representative of a larger decision to study caregivers together, as constituting a single household unit. In part, this approach draws on common knowledge of Oaxaca and many other Mexican settings about how individual decisions are oriented toward concern for the broader family. *Familismo* (family-centeredness) and *colectivismo* (collectivism) are but two related concepts that point to the experience of loyalty to one's family and broader community, a commitment to serve the larger group over oneself (Cervantes, 2008, p. 12; Keefe, Padilla, & Carlos, 1979; Smith-Morris et al., 2012). These orientations are dynamic and involve how individuals pool financial resources, living spaces, caregiving responsibilities, and moral strength to serve the larger social unit (Calzada, Tamis-LeMonda, & Yoshikawa, 2013). Individuals feel strengthened by these larger pools of support, and reciprocally experience obligations to contribute to them.[3] In Sergio's case, commitment to his family home is expressive of this felt responsibility; despite being an unmarried adult, he remains a contributing member of the household, supporting his parents and helping maintain their home. When or if he marries, social norms dictate that he redirects these responsibilities toward his new household, but he could continue to live with and provide support for his parents as well. For females, in contrast, norms dictate that married women relocate to live with husbands and in-laws. Yet regardless of these gender differences, all individuals in Teotitlán exist within larger social nexuses. Indeed, during the course of my fieldwork, I did not encounter a single individual who lived alone or with friends. All lived within family households. People seemed to take it as a given to support—and feel sustained by—the larger household, such that, to quote from another Oaxacan ethnographer, "to ignore the important role of the household [would be] to misunderstand how rural Oaxacans create their social universe" (J. Cohen, 2004, p. 23; see also Murphy & Stepick, 1991; Norget, 2006).[4]

This section is devoted toward describing the general nature of the Oaxacan caregiving household, tracing features that define households in the context of contemporary social change and beginning to put into focus how such change translates to the provision of elder care. All caregivers explained that they took on caregiving responsibilities because it was expected of them as proximate family members (that is, members who lived on or near the same property as forgetful elders) (see also Guarnaccia et al., 1992; Guarnaccia, 1998). Indeed, the very fact that there exists no Zapotec word for "caregiver" or a related concept demonstrates that providing care for members of the household is a presupposed feature of everyday life.[5] In Teotitlán as in most other Oaxacan settings, taking care of one's parents or one's spouse is simply what one does. Across my interviews with caregivers, nearly everyone responded with statements that they cared for elders "because he is my husband" or "because she is my mother." Caregivers adhered to relative social values about household and family cohesion, and they said that these efforts helped promote the larger family unit. Yet in the process of discussing how these values are upheld, caregivers also came to describe how contemporary features of social life have begun to challenge them.

An overview of the caregivers featured in this book illustrates how different family members have cobbled together household resources to jointly provide care for dependent elders. Table 1.1 identifies individual caregivers and basic identifying facts about their lives, respective households, and elders for whom they cared. As a whole, this table illustrates how different people come together for the provision of care, and how individuals act on behalf of the overall well-being of the larger household or family unit. This table also begins to introduce readers to the set of voices and the elders they cared for that comprise this larger study; it is my intention that readers continue to reference this table through the course of this book as additional households are presented. Even

Household	Caregivers	Age	Relationship to Elder	Elders	Age	Type of Forgetfulness	Level of Symptoms
1	Alberto Beatrice Cecilia	45 40 55	Son Daughter-in-law Daughter	Juana	75	Senile dementia	moderate-severe
2	Francisca Dominga	60 30	Sister Niece	Antonio	82	Stroke	moderate-severe
3	Mario Isabelle Graciela	40 35 75	Son Daughter-in-law Wife	Nicholas	80	Stroke	severe
4	Sergio Manuel Linda	30 45 70	Son Son Wife	Pedro	75	Undiagnosed progressive	moderate
5	Luis Laura	40 35	Son-in-law Daughter	Leticia	75	Undiagnosed progressive	mild
6	Juanita Anna	60 25	Wife Daughter	Jorge	70	Stroke	moderate-severe
7	Sophia	65	Wife	Vicente	77	Stroke	severe
8	Pablo Vanessa	40 35	N/A Niece-in-law	Maria	85	Alzheimer's disease	moderate-severe
9	Carlos Francisco Marta Jorge	75 50 45 20	Husband Son Daughter-in-law Grandson	Cynthia	70	Alzheimer's disease	severe

TABLE 1.1. Household Summary

through brief review of this table, and with but one exception, each caregiver spoke about his or her experience in the presence of other family members who also contributed to the provision of care. This is to say, caregiving is a family matter. Caregivers' ages spanned from early twenties to midseventies, showing how varying generational sectors and familial roles are involved in the caring process and work toward this broader social good. And, while some younger children were tangentially involved in caregiving, no household reported that these efforts were significant in maintaining responsibilities, presumably because children were expected to help with less-laborious domestic chores and to focus on school and other activities related to their development.

In Oaxaca these collectivist sensibilities extend beyond immediate family and household spheres and include individuals appropriated through *compadrazgo* (fictive kin) networks. This is a type of godparenthood where a respected community member takes on financial and moral responsibility for another family's children. This expands the scope of whom one can call upon as family, and the way in which Oaxacans can foster greater confidence and solidarity within the community (see Murphy & Stepick, 1991, pp. 149–53; Norget, 2006, pp. 47–49; Sault, 1985; Stephen, 2005, pp. 49–50). For example, during my first experience at a wedding in Teotitlán, I was impressed to learn that although most guests were family members, nearly 500 people (a tenth of the 5,500-member community) were present. Through this and other interactions, I came to realize the impressive lengths that family networks reached. Indeed, in the context of this social setting, one of the most confusing hypothetical questions I initially posed to Alex was, what would happen if an elder did not have any family support. Alex and every other Teotiteco I had questioned responded exactly the same: "Your question doesn't make sense here." In Teotitlán there is a common understanding that every individual exists within a larger family network, and it is inconceivable that a person would find him- or herself without recourse to social support.

Familial relationships are strong in Oaxaca, but the reality is more complicated. Sergio and his family discussed how their parents have their own godchildren and a robust compadrazgo network, but then stated that these family visits have become more of a formality than a tangible source of help. "They can't be obliged to come," his brother said, and reflected on how help from other, more distant members of compadrazgo networks was more limited than he would have hoped. Similarly, Sergio and Manuel also discussed how other individuals in their immediate family who did not live with their parents also did not distribute caregiving responsibilities equally. They mentioned their sister, Janet, who lived in Teotitlán on different property with her husband and family. They described how Janet's visits were helpful in taking on supplemental responsibilities like reading to Pedro and distracting him from agitation. But the family told me that the infrequency of these visits limited the effects of Janet's good intentions. Other forms of absence further challenged the apparent cohesiveness of Sergio's household. While Manuel called Teotitlán his primary home, he visited California every few months to sell rugs and maintain other business, and had another brother who primarily lived in California and returned to Teotitlán a few times a year, less often than the family would prefer. At one point, when Manuel talked about this brother, he said, "It definitely affects us [not having all our family in one place] because not all of us are taking care of him. They don't live here and don't really know what's going on."

This point is not solely representative of shifting household trends, but of larger ones throughout the community marked by migration. More individuals are pursuing economic opportunities away from Oaxaca, which fragments households and families. Though it is difficult to accurately measure migration trends, a survey conducted by Rafael Reyes Morales and Alicia Silvia Gijón Cruz (2002) estimates that the average number of persons who had emigrated from Teotitlán in early 2000s was 0.57 people per household, or approximately 500 individuals per the 950 households in the community (p. 20). These are only estimates, however, and my anecdotal experience suggests that these rates may be higher. Indeed, while these numbers speak to the significant social fragmentation associated with migration, evidence from surrounding communities further puts into focus how transborder realities impact local household cohesion and provision of elder care. An article in *Síntesis*, a regional Oaxacan newspaper, reports that 5 to 10 percent of all elderly patients in hospitals came because they had been abandoned and lack social support because of migration (Jiménez, 2014). And, in other Oaxacan settings like Santo Domingo Tonalá, there now exists an NGO providing daycare (consisting primarily of social support) to elders who have few remaining family members in the community.[6]

But Teotitecos insist that these systemic changes are not occurring in their own community. Indeed, similar to the response to my question about elders lacking social support, locals consistently stated that elders do not need to worry about growing dependent. This proved true during my fieldwork, but that statement and response were far more complicated than the simplicity they implied. To consider another household, during my interview with Pablo and Vanessa, I came to realize that some households might care for elders who are not in their immediate families because there is no one else available to provide care. Pablo and Vanessa are a married couple with their own children who decided to do an *obra de caridad* (act of charity) by caring for an elder who had nowhere else to live. The elder had migrated to Mexico City and, upon returning to Teotitlán as a widow in old age, was denied care by immediate family members. Pablo and Vanessa assumed responsibility for this elder because they realized no one else would. The case of Pablo and Vanessa illustrates that sometimes social ideals do not translate to local realities: elder care is not always maintained because of the family cohesiveness that local traditions dictate, and the distribution of caregiving responsibilities is impacted by larger social circumstances.

Migration and related shifts in social practices impact the distribution of caregiving responsibilities; whereas some family members migrate away from the community to economically provide for the household, remaining proximate members respond to fill the "care slot" caused by their absence (Leinaweaver, 2010; Parreñas, 2015; Scott, 2012; Yarris, 2017). In Teotitlán, with such emphasis on household cohesion, different individuals jointly contribute to filling these absences: Sergio, with his parents because he was unmarried; Manuel, in a separate household on the same property with his own family; and Linda, continuing to support her husband alongside the help she received from her two adult children.

Talking about these household realities also highlighted the broader economics of caregiving responsibilities, how care is circulated among family members across political borders, financial and social structures, and cultural expectations (Baldassar, Baldock, & Wilding, 2007; Baldassar & Merla, 2013). In this perspective care is not only defined by hands-on embodied work, but also involves economic, moral, and social support that can be exchanged across borders. This is helpful in accounting for the remittances sent from migrants to financially support caregivers at home, as well as for the exchange of goods like clothes, and for the moral support provided over the internet and phone. Through these contributions, absent family members are able to participate in caregiving efforts and have a sense of involvement in the household, transcending borders that physically separate them (Bryceson & Vuorela, 2003). But Sergio's family and all the households I studied made a distinction between this form of help and the embodied, proximate care that they provided on a daily level. Manuel made this observation when he reflected on how his living in a separate household from Sergio and Linda impacted how he was able to care. "It's not the same for me as my brother," Manuel said. It matters that a person knows what it is like to be summoned on a regular basis, and knows that another's well-being depends on these efforts.

These contemporary transborder realities, paired with the immediate demands of caregiving, prompt family members to come together in other unexpected ways. They challenge cultural and gendered norms about who is expected to provide care in a setting where those human resources are increasingly harder to come by. Indeed, one of the more surprising overall experiences while conducting this study was encountering so many men who were not only involved but claimed primary responsibility for elders' care: overall, 40 percent of the caregivers were men, comprising nearly half of total participants (see chart 1.1). This ran against what I read in the literature and what other locals who were not involved in care predicted, that women would hold primary caregiving responsibilities (Ayalon & Huyck, 2002; Henderson & Guitierrez-Mayka, 1992). Like other Oaxacan settings, in Teotitlán domestic labor is often classified by gender. Typically, men are expected to provide financial support through weaving production and sales, small-scale farming, and fulfillment of *cargos*. In contrast, although women have begun to take on "untraditional" roles like weaving production and sales as well as cargo services, they are traditionally tasked with carrying out domestic chores, including preparation of food, cleaning, and raising children (see Stephen, 2005).[7] Throughout Teotitlán and Oaxaca, residents implicitly held caregiving as a task designated to women of the household. Those who provided care on a daily basis challenged this norm.

In addition to gender, across households there were other patterns about which members assumed primary caregiving responsibilities and how they were distributed. Four households identified one person who held more responsibilities than all other members, while the remainder of participants said that caregiving responsibility was divided equally with another or all members of the family. Most often, adult children assumed care for their parents: 36 percent of all caregivers were adult biological children, and 18 percent were adult in-law children, which together comprises 54 percent of this study's total participants (see chart 1.2). Again, these often crossed gender lines, though there were

CHART 1.1. Gender Among Caregivers

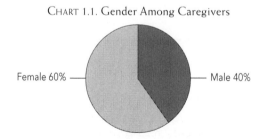

CHART 1.2. Caregivers' Relationships to Elders

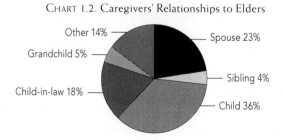

notable gender differences. When adult sons were primary caregivers, they typically held this role in support of their own biological parents. This stands in comparison to adult daughters, who tended to hold primary caregiving responsibilities more often for their in-laws (with whom they relocated to live after getting married). When there existed a spouse of the dependent elder, he or she was consistently involved in caregiving, either equally sharing or primarily holding responsibility.

These observations more broadly illustrate the novel ways members of households come together to respond to elders' needs and family absences. On the one hand, caregivers continue to prioritize the household as the primary social unit. Households are established on the basis of marriage arrangements, with married women relocating to live with in-law families and men continuing to live with their own parents. Yet while these norms are upheld, others have begun to change. In the context of greater domestic fragmentation, caregiving responsibilities traverse normative gender divisions and generate novel social arrangements.

THE "PROBLEM" OF AGING IN TEOTITLÁN

While household and family structure help contextualize the voices of this study, equally important are the current perceptions of aging itself. These perceptions are on public display. To start, the *greca* provides initial clues about how elders are viewed as an integral part of the lifecycle and intergenerational continuity. Cast in the concrete of main streets and woven in countless rugs, the greca is one of the most common symbols of regional Zapotec culture. It is traced back to the stone walls of surrounding archeological ruins, a pattern of five descending steps that, at its termination, rotates direction and initiates another set of steps (see figure 1.1). Each step represents a different stage of the lifecycle, while its transformation into another greca is a symbol for death and intergenerational continuity. The implicit metaphor is that while aging represents the termination of one lifecycle, an elder's place in society and their knowledge of tradition helps foster continuity for future generations.

Yet depictions of the community implying a repetitive reproduction of values stand in juxtaposition to others that point toward how values are dynamically regenerated. Alongside the concrete grecas at the intersection of Teotitlán's two principal roads exists a series of hand-painted murals depicting various public health initiatives. There are murals to promote awareness of dengue fever, the right to receive sexual education, the dangers of domestic violence, and, within

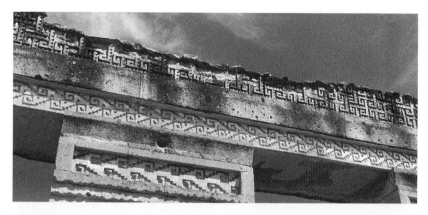

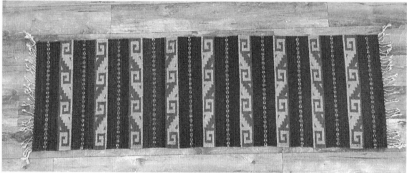

FIGS. 1.1a & 1.1b. Two depictions of *grecas*. The first is a photograph of Zapotec ruins in Mitla, and the second a rug woven in Teotitlán. *Photographs by the author.*

this series, one will also find a statement on aging (see figure 1.2). In contrast to the greca, this mural suggests that simplified depictions of aging are actually situated more in shades of gray. The mural's red title announces "Seniors" [*Adultos Mayores*] and underneath states: "You're Never too Old to Surprise Yourself" [*No Hay Edad Para Sorprenderse a Uno Mismo*]. In the middle there is a large illustration of a yellow pyramid, with one side that specifies factors leading to successful aging (balanced diet, exercise, social support, and health), and another side that lists inhibiting factors (addiction, self-neglect, lack of exercise, and poor diet). Atop the pyramid stand two elders holding hands, providing an image of what health looks like in old age—and whose Caucasian skin speaks to this issue being framed as a modern one. Underneath the illustration reads: "The Problem of Old Age Isn't Age Itself" (*El Problema de la Vejez No Es la Edad*).[8]

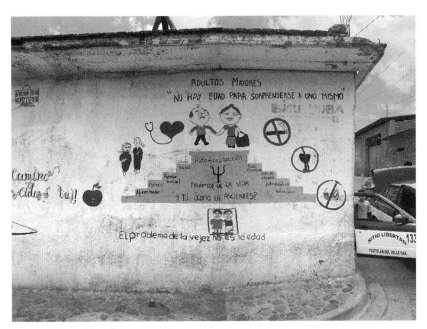

FIG. 1.2. *The Problem of Aging* mural. *Photograph by the author, digitally edited by Michelle Nermon to remove a center-standing telephone pole.*

Of course, by stating that age is not "the problem of old age" the mural suggests that there *is* a problem to be dealt with. It speaks to the growing problems faced by elder Teotitecos and tries to promote an alternative vision that promises greater self-fulfillment, social integration, and novel life experiences. Though the mural makes a call to action for elders to improve their lives, it also implicitly speaks to the broader Teotiteco population by offering a statement that being old is not a disability, and that elders are capable of contributing to the community. Yet given how much elders *are* heralded in this setting, it is curious to come across this public health initiative to contest ageist assumptions. I began to wonder: did this campaign lack an understanding of the local Teotiteco community, or was there some truth here about aging that the community needed to address?

A closer look at two demographic patterns helps provide context. The first concerns the overall presence of elders in society, both in number and proportion of the population. Teotitlán's percentage of elders (defined as over age 60) has risen from 8 percent in 1980 to 15 percent in 2010. This stands in contrast to the national average in 2010, where people over 60 comprised 9.1 percent of the total population. The overall increased proportion of elders in Mexican society reflects a national demographic transformation: whereas in 2000 there were currently nine children for every elder, in 2050 there will be an equal number of elders to children, and elders will represent one-fifth of the total population (Jackson, 2005). Mexico's increased longevity is a result of public health campaigns initially launched during the middle of the twentieth century to better control infectious diseases, meet nutritional needs, and improve medical care (Haber et al., 2008, pp. 163–71). These efforts, coupled with lowered mortality and fertility rates, family planning campaigns, and promotion of contraceptives, gave rise to a population that is quickly aging (Wong & Palloni, 2009, pp. 236–37).[9]

A more focused perspective of this trend within Teotitlán reveals how remarkable it is on a local level. From 1930 (when census data is first available) to 2010, Teotitlán exhibited a 133 percent growth in the overall population, with 76 percent increase in youths (aged 0–19), 133 percent gain in adults (aged 20–59), and a disproportional 644 percent increase in elders (aged 60+) (see chart 1.3).[10] Or, stated differently, whereas in 1930 there were 8.6 youths for every elder, this ratio progressively dropped such that by 2010 there were only two youths for every elder. These patterns indicate that elders are significantly more prevalent than ever before in Teotitlán's demographic history.

The second change concerns differences within the aging population itself: more people are living longer, reaching ages that were previously unimaginable. Whereas in 1921 the national life expectancy was 32.9 years, by 2010 life expectancy became 74.5 years (77.4 for women and 71.7 for men) (INEGI, 2015; see also Partida-Bush, 2005).[11] In Teotitlán during the 1930s, only two individuals reached 80 years or more (constituting less than 0.01 percent of the total population), whereas the number of "old-elders" has steadily risen such that by 2010, there were 175 individuals (comprising 3.1 percent of the population).

Together, these two demographic patterns suggest that Teotitlán is encountering new realities about old age: elders are simultaneously more prevalent in society *and* are aging into later decades than ever before. These changes have undoubtedly ushered in others as well. There is now greater prevalence of illness associated with old age, economic and physical dependence, and related difficulties participating in the community. And, while there are overall more elders in need of greater care, there are fewer adults and youths able to meet their needs. Lower fertility rates, improved life expectancies, and migration patterns have all contributed toward this trend.

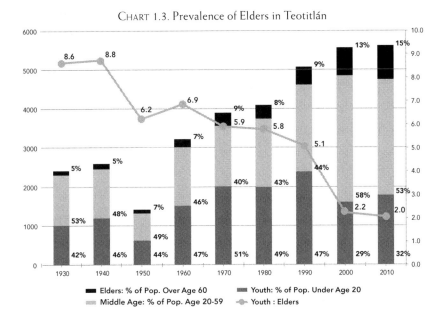

CHART 1.3. Prevalence of Elders in Teotitlán

These patterns help contextualize how aging comes to represent—and be constituted within—a specific constellation of social issues. It is not just the fact that elders are becoming more prevalent and growing older, but that these demographic trends are interpreted and experienced in a way specific to Teotitlán. They are understood as instances that put into question how the community will support and maintain itself in the context of changes surrounding it.

The way age is understood as an issue specific to Teotitlán is expressive of the broader point about how age can mean something different across social settings, depending on time and place. This is a lesson drawn from the social constructionists, who remind us that social categories like age and illness are not fixed, but rather constituted within broader social factors that always fluctuate and reconstitute their meanings (Berger & Luckmann, 1967; Cole & Ray, 2010; Estes, 1979; Gergen, 2009; Gubrium & Holstein, 2000; Parker, 1998).[12] For example, it is telling that during the sixteenth and early seventeenth centuries, people in the United States extolled elders precisely for their fragility and dependency—features then interpreted to characterize mankind's ultimate relationship with God. Later, during the eighteenth and nineteenth centuries, these ideals gave way to the pursuit of capitalistic enterprise, passion for material wealth, and personal autonomy. Aging subsequently became a symbol of moral failure, representing the "old world" of patriarchy and revealing the limitations of self-governance (Cole, 1992). Appreciating how old age is constructed within broader social dynamics is not just an intellectual point, but one that directly shapes many of the assumptions about and responses to it.[13]

In Teotitlán, social constructionism helps put into focus what it means for elders to increase in prevalence and age, and how these meanings disclose broader concerns within this larger social setting. Historically, the people of the clouds—the Zapotec—were people who venerated elders because they represented tradition and knowledge about how to maintain it. In the colonial era, the period from which we have some of the first written records of language practices in Teotitlán, the Zapotec word for elder was *penicòlà*.[14] Given what we know of royal ancestor worship at this period in history, it seems likely that this word connoted something close to a person's authority and wisdom of local tradition. Today, the Zapotec word for elder—*bengul*—literally means "person who is mature in age." As there are no gender pronouns in Zapotec, this word refers to the aged maturity found among both men and women. Most often, the word connotes a sense of prestige and respect on the basis of elders' accumulation of life experience, much like the word "president" does. Such perceptions coalesce around the Zapotec notion of *respet* (respect, a Spanish cognate from the word *respeto*). Respet is a concept that refers to the amount of authority and honor a person is endowed by other members of the community. Respected individuals are greeted with a distinct handshake and spoken to with different pronouns and verb conjugations. As one adult explained, "Elders have more experience than we have had. . . . In our community, they're the ones that are respected the most. Because of our customs and you perhaps know it because in a *fiesta* they're the first ones to be called on. So they're the most important part of the community. And they deserve respect."

Such statements were an anthem during my research. But while elders were commonly said to have earned respect through their life experiences, locals' use of another word—*bingul*—further complicates this claim. In contrast to the word bengul (person mature with age), the Zapotec word bingul translates to mean "a younger person who is mature."[15] When this latter word is used in the context of aging, it creates a distinction between age and authority: bengul is then used to refer simply to an "elder," in contrast to bingul, which is used to refer to a "younger mature person." Each household has its own bingul, the person who makes decisions, is sought for advice, and in general holds highest authority. Indeed, while most elders would be considered a bingul with authority and respect, locals hastened to clarify that sometimes this does not always apply. Some households like Manuel's lived with no elder, so the next person to demonstrate knowledge is considered the representative bingul. And, more to the point of this book, locals also said that some elders might lose their accumulated life wisdom and authority owing to poor health and lack of insight. The implicit authority and respect associated with old age becomes rendered in a new light. Indeed, these semantic subtleties further point toward how aging has taken on varying meanings, and what is at stake in elders' forgetfulness.

It seems like an often-repeated trope across time and place that elders have lost the respect traditionally given to them, but in Teotitlán this complaint seems to carry tangible social weight. In addition to semantic differences about aging, many caregivers described how elders might not always be seen through the respect and authority their age would typically confer. Juanita is a caregiver who reflected on how elders are sometimes criticized because they cannot participate in society like their neighbors. "There are people that treat elders with respect," she said, "and there are others that criticize elders. And there are people that ask themselves why some elders go out in public and participate in fiestas if they can barely walk." Similarly Graciela, another caregiver, reflected on her own experience being an elder in the community when she said, "The way we grew up back then is a lot different compared to now. I think people just don't understand us [elders] sometimes. And that's my personal point of view—it's that people get tired of us." Other caregivers described this change in more drastic terms. Francisca and Dominga are two caregivers from a different household who reflected on how some Teotiteco elders have become objects of ridicule because they are not perceived to be "normal" (using the Zapotec adjective *sro*, which varyingly means "normal," "good," or "pretty"). Dominga went on to say, "I think people nowadays think poorly not only towards ill people, but elders as well. They don't value them as human beings but rather look at them based on what's wrong with them. . . . They focus on their [productive] capacity. . . . People tend to think more for themselves than to empathize." Many Teotitecos would take objection to this statement and claim that elders continue to be respected, and most of the observations made during my fieldwork align with this objection. However, beyond what I came to discover through the important exceptions that age-related forgetfulness engendered, there exists tangible evidence that representations of aging have begun to shift.

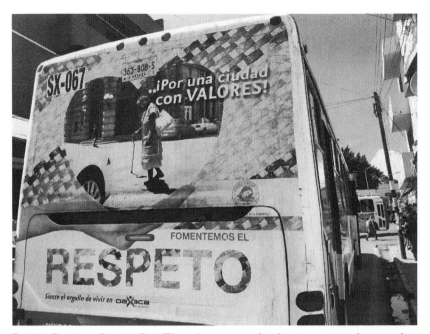

FIG. 1.3. *Respeto* in Oaxaca City. This advertisement for the importance of respect for elders was found on the back of a bus in Oaxaca City. Again illustrating how urban settings are linked to a perceived of lack of respect, this image is also interesting for how Caucasian hands are framing the image. It shows how social campaigns about maintaining respect are linked with notions about modernity and global influence. *Photograph by the author.*

In addition to these perspectives, other systemic changes have occurred. One involves the political authority typically allotted to elders within the cargo system—a system that is justified as preserving tradition by allotting political power to elders who, in their lifetimes, ascend to posts with increasing prestige. But in Teotitlán and across Oaxaca, the cargo system has slowly transformed such that younger candidates are holding prestigious positions that were traditionally allotted to elders. This was first observed decades ago when Kate Young (1976) described the case of village elders in another Oaxacan community who had lost social standing to hold public office to members of the community that instead emphasized youth, accumulation of wealth, and engagement with national culture—features that are considered opposed to maintenance of local identity and tradition. And more recently, Mary Gagnier de Mendoza (2005) has described public celebrations of events in Teotitlán like Holy Thursday, and parenthetically mentions that the role traditionally prescribed to a cohort of respected elders to reenact the story of Christ was given to younger community members (p. 91). Though subtle, these social changes help further contextualize the way in which traditional roles prescribed to elders have recently begun to evolve.

Indeed, these broader social changes in the community show how new features of old age are understood in the context of larger social issues. Migration, alternative lifestyles based on capitalism and social independence, and the impact of other foreign influences simultaneously highlight how social arrangements in Teotitlán are being regenerated, and how the community negotiates to maintain cohesion in this context. Elders are at the center of this social dynamic. As they tend to be viewed as sources of intergenerational continuity, elders' difficulties upholding that image *qua* illness and related dependencies are representative of what is at stake in a community attempting to maintain a sense of cohesion. Moreover, the very symptoms of forgetfulness further put into question the authority that elders are typically endowed. Like Sergio who described the challenge of respecting his father whose disruptive behaviors called respect into question, all of the caregivers for this study discussed the complicated reality of maintaining respect for forgetful elders while recognizing that forgetful elders seem to have lost the authority that is conferred with their advanced age. Caregivers noted that forgetful elders are no longer asked to give advice at weddings, not the first to enter the altar room, and not called upon to arbitrate disagreements. As one caregiver observed of his forgetful mother, "During a fiesta or with relatives, now it's very seldom when her opinion matters." Such individuals are referred to through the term *bengul*—"elder"—in contrast to the way their age might otherwise mark their standing as bingul. This shift and its subsequent social implications are the topic of the following section.

FORGETTING ALZHEIMER'S IN TEOTITLÁN

One of the most informative ways I came to appreciate what age-related forgetfulness means in Teotitlán was through inquiring about the severest form of it. Sergio and his family said they had heard of Alzheimer's disease and knew that one of its primary symptoms involves the way elders remain sedentary and stare. Manuel indexed this knowledge through reference to popular depictions of Ronald Reagan he had encountered while living in California. "Didn't Ronald

Reagan have Alzheimer's? The ex-president of the United States. That's how we heard of Alzheimer's [for the first time], and that's how I saw what people with Alzheimer's look like. They just sit down, just like objects. [Reagan] was just sitting and staring." Sergio and his family discussed how they knew about Alzheimer's and were even told by their local dentist that Pedro's forgetfulness might owe to it. But they repeatedly expressed this view to be mistaken. Manuel said, "I think that if he had that disease, he wouldn't be able to do anything else, because . . . people with Alzheimer's are just gone, just sitting and forget about everything."

Yet despite claiming that Pedro did not have Alzheimer's, it was striking how accounts of Pedro's behavior seemed to match what they described of it. Sergio and his family described Pedro mindlessly staring in numerous contexts, such as finding him looking indiscriminately at walls or off toward a distant a horizon. And, at one point, Linda described how Pedro's tendency to stare made every-day caregiving tasks like bathing significantly more difficult:

> When [I finally manage to get him to] shower, I give him his clothes. But when I give them to him he won't put them on. He'll just take them to dirty baskets. [So a week ago] I went to get another pair of pants, and then he sat and started staring at the pants, checking out everything about them. He just looked at every part of the pants, as if they weren't well made or something. And then he folded them, and put them in another drawer. . . . And also two days ago the same thing happened. He was told to shower and he was just sitting down and staring at his pants. And then he showered. Afterward I told him to put on his clothes again, but he did the same thing, just stared at his pants. And every time they ask him to put it on, he won't do it.

Such descriptions were helpful to appreciate this family's caregiving experience, but they also provide important insight into larger social understandings of Alzheimer's disease, age-related forgetfulness more generally, and the broader stigma associated with these conditions. They demonstrate how households like Sergio's contest and avoid understanding elders as having Alzheimer's and provide clues toward how age-related forgetfulness is representative of concerns about broader social change.

I noted similar observations in other corners of my fieldwork. For example, on the front page of NOTICIAS, one of the state's most circulated and respected newspapers, I encountered a curious article on Alzheimer's disease that further contextualized local understandings. In bold capital letters the title announced:

20 ALZHEIMER'S CASES HAVE BEEN DETECTED [20 CASOS DE ALZHEIMER SE HAN DETECT-ADO] (Chavela, 2014). Although the Mexican press is known for its sensationalism, I was nevertheless struck by the way Alzheimer's was portrayed as an epidemic, in language that was remarkably similar to current stories on the Ebola virus. The article described that the State of Oaxaca is proposing to follow Mexico City, which has implemented a bracelet program to locate and return the growing number of older adults who wander from their homes. The article explained, "Many with it [Alzheimer's] leave their homes and go astray" (*Muchas de ellas salen de sus hogares y se extravían*).[16] It further illustrated the difficulty of detecting Alzheimer's because symptoms are often attributable to other conditions, and it stated that the disease is irreversible and progressive (*irreversible y progresiva*) and compromises an elder's ability to carry out basic functions. The article then concluded with suggestions for treating Alzheimer's, with tips for how to manage behavioral problems through modifying the home environment and "offering help to the family who suffers the most" (*ofrecer apoyo a la familia que es la que sufre más*). Both the NOTICIAS article and Sergio's family perception reveal the nuanced ways Alzheimer's is understood locally as an age-related disease that is rare and threatening, perceived in context to its disruption of family and broader social dynamics.

There was a common finding throughout my fieldwork where doctors, traditional healers, municipal clerks, and laypersons all told me that they had heard of Alzheimer's, but believed it was nonexistent in Teotitlán. Indeed, one local physician even told me that he knew of a village near the coast that had a high prevalence of Alzheimer's, but could not explain why he did not know of a single case in Teotitlán. As I came to learn, Alzheimer's was held to not exist because, in part, it is locally perceived as an illness that arises in a different psychosocial environment. As one acquaintance told me, "People do not have Alzheimer's disease because they don't need to worry about paying the rent, and other [forms of] stress experienced over there [for example, other metropolitan settings like Oaxaca City and the United States]." Alzheimer's was understood as a modern condition that occurred because of stresses associated with nontraditional ways of living, experienced by migrants who jettison local ways of life and locals who embrace foreign values. "This is a very new thing," one caregiver said of his wife diagnosed with Alzheimer's. "To me diabetes is a new disease. All those other diseases are new too, like cancer. Back in the days, there were no such things. People used to die, but due to other illnesses." Like Sergio's household, individuals wanted to believe Alzheimer's did not exist because of its negative association to modern lifestyles and, of those who knew otherwise, there was strong reluctance to speak about it.

To be sure, there are other reasons for why Alzheimer's is said to not exist locally. While there are more pressing medical issues like dengue fever and diabetes, another reason is the reality that there is little industry surrounding Alzheimer's. The economic stakeholders that have helped make Alzheimer's into such a publicly recognized illness within the United States do not exist in Oaxaca with the same influence.[17] This is despite the relative accessibility of medical care—Teotitlán has a local medical clinic, and consultations are subsidized to $20 pesos (U.S. $1.25), plus costs for filling prescriptions. Yet a scantly existing age-related pharmaceutical industry means that physicians are less invested to diagnose cases.[18] And, in comparison to the United States, where a diagnosis is accompanied by other options like professional nursing care and retirement homes, in Oaxaca these options seem to be a distant vision. There are three nursing homes in the state, two publicly funded and another privately funded. Though some residents of these homes have dementia, these facilities are not designed to provide this type of care, and specifically require that elders have the cognitive capacity to self-admit to become a resident.[19] These structural facts indicate how Alzheimer's disease in Oaxaca is situated among fewer economic stakeholders, leading to a smaller number of people invested in prompting awareness.

Indeed, I initially arrived to Oaxaca intent to ask locals about Alzheimer's disease, only to realize that we were adopting two different meanings of the same word. I assumed that my understanding of Alzheimer's was standard across cultures, and that it would be possible to inquire about it locally with mutual understanding. But this "category fallacy" reified my own clinical knowledge onto another setting and put into focus nuanced differences in the local meanings attributed to age-related forgetfulness (Kleinman, 1988b). This became apparent with Alberto, Beatrice, and Cecilia, another caregiving household that reflected on how a diagnosis of senile dementia was not alarming, compared to Alzheimer's: "Well, when they [the doctors] told us [our mother had senile dementia] . . . we were worried because we didn't know what it was. But when they explained it, we didn't take it seriously because what the doctor said that what was serious is Alzheimer's disease." Throughout my fieldwork I came to recognize that there were two different forms of progressive age-related forgetfulness. In contrast to Alzheimer's, senile dementia is a diagnostic term used more frequently in Oaxaca, known as a condition where elders progressively forget but remain capable of interacting and functioning in their environment at a basic level.[20] Alzheimer's disease, on the other hand, is perceived to be a more severe form of forgetting, where the individual is unaware of his or her surroundings, and unable to participate in social life.

This basic distinction also involved how forgetfulness is linguistically differentiated into distinct types. In Zapotec there is a distinction between *rienlá'az*, which refers to the forgetfulness of objects, and *raguenlá'az*, which is the forgetting of a person. When the type of forgetfulness associated with Alzheimer's was described, it was almost always indexed to this latter term. Indeed, while locals make this distinction and use it to avoid acknowledging the presence of Alzheimer's, they also seemed to intuit how a less alarming type of forgetfulness might progress into one more serious. This included cases of senile dementia and forgetfulness caused by stroke. As will be seen throughout this book, at stake in forgetfulness involves the ways families and, by extension, the larger community are able to maintain a sense of cohesion. Hence, and in contrast to settings that prioritize memory for the way it allows people to function independently, in Teotitlán memory serves the function of keeping individuals together, with forgetfulness representing a threat to that value. As Beatrice came to say of the importance of memory as she observed the forgetfulness of her mother-in-law, "It's important because we have kids and I have a husband. I can't even imagine that I could forget that I have children or forget that I have a husband."

Before further discussing this perception, it is helpful to pause to consider how the meaning of forgetfulness and Alzheimer's disease might vary not only in places like Oaxaca that appropriate biomedical information from afar, but also within the United States and other "Western" settings where that information is generated from within. As Atwood Gaines (1987) was the first to argue in the 1980s, Alzheimer's is an explicit "Western concept" with specific Western values, rooted in a culture that prioritizes cognition over relational capacities and autonomy over collective functioning.

It may appear odd to claim that Alzheimer's—a specific neuropathology defined by the presence of amyloid plaques and neurofibrillary tangles—can be said to mean something different, depending on the surrounding environment. Indeed, the estimated prevalence of dementia (with Alzheimer's being the most common type) is roughly similar across global regions: for those age sixty-plus, rates range from 4 to 8 percent, but within this spectrum Latin American settings score on the higher end (Prince et al., 2015). To be sure, the neuropathology associated with Alzheimer's does not change across time and place so much as the interpretation of what it signifies. This idea is perhaps best explained through Ian Hacking's (1986) concept of "dynamic nominalism," a variant of social constructionism, which posits that kinds of people (for example, elders with Alzheimer's) come into existence at the same moment as there appear respective kinds of categories (for example, Alzheimer's disease) used to make sense of them (see Lock [2007] for further development of this concept with regard to Alzheimer's). Dynamic nominalism acknowledges that there are underlying neurological features that help account for what Alzheimer's is, but places greater emphasis on how neuropathology is understood and categorized into a discrete social phenomenon that can be called "a case of Alzheimer's disease." Moreover, it points to the ways that categories—like pathological and normal aging—are not static, but subject to the way societies varyingly define them. To use the title of Hacking's essay, this is the process of "making up people."

Dynamic nominalism is strikingly relevant to appreciate the history of Alzheimer's disease. After all, during the first half of the twentieth century, Alzheimer's was considered an insignificant disease that affected a very small number of people. This opinion, featured in the first reported case, extends to 1906, when German psychiatrist Alois Alzheimer studied the now famous fifty-one-year-old woman who displayed symptoms of progressive dementia, hallucinations, and delusions. Alzheimer hypothesized that the clinical symptoms he had studied were a consequence of the neuropathology he had discovered during autopsy that revealed senile plaques and twisted bundles of neurofibrillary tangles.[21] Yet what is so fascinating about this early history is that the psychiatric community was interested in this case *not* because of senility in itself, but rather because senility manifested in a woman considered too young to develop it. Alzheimer believed that the original significance of his discovery was that people younger than previously recognized could become senile. Alzheimer called these cases "atypical forms of senile dementia," implying that there is a "typical" form of senile dementia expected to occur among older populations (quoted in Dillman, 2000, p. 136).

The original understanding of Alzheimer's disease as something that affects people in their fifties—and senility being a normal feature of aging—persisted until the 1970s, with age of onset serving as the only distinguishing criterion.[22] Yet even today, as Alzheimer's has gained a firm foothold in U.S. political and social discourse, there remains ambiguity concerning its underlying cause. We have difficulty distinguishing the neuropathology associated with Alzheimer's from the standard course of aging. Moreover, the same plaques and tangles definitive of Alzheimer's are found among most aging persons, irrespective of whether or not they exhibit cognitive impairment (Xekardaki et al., 2015).[23] And some researchers even hypothesize, in contrast to the dominant opinion that plaques and tangles are the cause of clinical symptoms, that these neurological processes may actually be reparative or compensatory reactions (Glass & Arnold, 2012). This clinical ambiguity is a resounding theme of Margaret Lock's book *The Alzheimer's Conundrum* (2013), where leading neurologists, geneticists, epidemiologists, and psychiatrists are all shown to express uncertainty about neurological substrates of Alzheimer's, challenging us to "confront head-on the ontological question of what exactly is [Alzheimer's]" (p. 2).

I present this literature not to dismiss the dreadful significance of Alzheimer's or the positive impact empirical science might have toward its cure. Rather, these uncertainties help contextualize how Alzheimer's meaning is constituted within a broader cultural outlook.[24] Indeed, the commonly embraced idea that Alzheimer's is "a death that leaves the body behind" is only intelligible within a "hypercognitive" culture that equates selfhood with cognition (Post, 2000). In Japan, senility is considered a threat to cultural expectations to remain economically productive (Traphagan, 1998); in Vietnam, individuals have been shown to be indifferent regarding the development of dementia symptoms in later life (Braun & Browne, 1998); in India, cultural anxieties contextualize focus on elders' symptoms of anger over ones of cognitive decline (L. Cohen, 1998); in Brazil, senile forgetfulness is distinguished from a positive capacity to forget sociocultural stress (Leibing, 2002); and, in U.S. Native American settings, while forgetfulness is considered normal, concomitant psychotic symptoms are understood to be evidence of communication with the supernatural world (Henderson & Henderson, 2002). These varying perceptions of the same clinical entity serve to remind us that surrounding values and social circumstances matter—that selfhood is not necessarily equated with cognition. Indeed, in the United States, Alzheimer's is so terrifying because it hits the core of what it means to be a person in this setting—so much that Jesse Ballenger (2006) cogently writes that Alzheimer's "haunt[s] the landscape of the self-made man" (p. 9).

A respective lesson can be drawn of local understandings in Teotitlán.[25] In addition to Sergio's observation that Alzheimer's is a condition where elders sit and stare, he and his family also associated general instances of forgetfulness to be caused by the stress associated to modern, nontraditional lifestyles. The family reflected on how throughout their lives they had never encountered another elder who exhibited behaviors similar to those they encountered with Pedro. Manuel tried to account for forgetfulness through contrasting levels of stress and social circumstance:

> Nowadays, [forgetfulness] happens because a lot of people are stressed. And back then people lived a more tranquil life. Their lives back then were very calm. But now, these days, it's crazy [*Manuel gestures to his head*]. Nowadays people think way too much. And back in those days, people who lived here [in Teotitlán] were self-sufficient. And today, we have to work to get other goods. And so, all of this stresses people out.

Manuel's comments further illustrate how stress associated with social change is the cause for elders' forgetfulness. These are stresses related to absent family members owing to migration, focus on capital gain, and other forms of social tension viewed to be challenging how the community maintains a sense of cohesion. Manuel's comments illustrate how age-related forgetfulness is situated within this dynamic, but it also shows what is at stake for people to acknowledge that life has become stressful. Immediately following Manuel's observations about modern stress, his mother Linda comments, "He actually lived a very tranquil life." And Manuel adds: "Yes, he had a tranquil life. . . . That's why we wonder why he's the way he is. Because I see other people that have more kids and a lot more things to worry about. And so I don't know why [he's this way]." While Sergio and his family simultaneously understand age-related forgetfulness in the context of stress and social change, they resist attributing this understanding to make sense of the forgetfulness they encounter at home. Forgetfulness is suggestive of the stress involved in pursuit of a different, modern lifestyle—something that most locals seem to want to avoid acknowledging in their own lives.

Yet the alleged difference between local culture and what resides "over there" is a much more contested issue. While Teotitecos claim that Alzheimer's disease is something that manifests outside the community, the cases I came to gather of age-related forgetfulness show how locals are encountering notable exceptions. Indeed, Teotitlán has and continues to socially evolve such that what is outside the community is, in many respects, already a part of local reality (Stephen, 2007; Wood, 2000). Yes, in Teotitlán individuals do not need to pay rent, and yes, life is qualitatively slower, with fewer forms of stress associated with a "modern" lifestyle. But as Sergio and all other locals attest, life has become more stressful, and these features of contemporary life are linked to larger social trends concerning migration, capital pursuits, and related systemic change. In this way, the belief that Alzheimer's and other forms of age-related forgetfulness manifest outside Teotitlán begins to take on a different meaning. It provides more information about what is occurring on a local level than what is viewed to be happening outside. It shows, following Susan Sontag (2001), how illnesses are so often imbued with moral claims. And, it reveals the segre-social dimensions of how illness impacts everyday life: age-related forgetfulness is a symbol of the perceived difference between local and foreign lifestyles, standing as the looming threat of modernity over the preservation of local tradition.

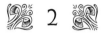

Idioms of Distress

SYMPTOMS AND ETIOLOGIES OF
PROGRESSIVE FORGETFULNESS

Overnight Cecilia boils and soaks *maize* from her family's section of communal farmland, and in the morning, she gathers it to be transported to the *molino* to be ground. At 55 years old, Cecilia is unmarried and so continues to live with Juana, her widowed mother. Her brother, Alberto, lives in an adjacent home with his own family on the same family property. In the morning he exits to the shared family courtyard, followed by his wife, Beatrice. The three gather briefly in the space that joins their respective homes, a plot of unpaved, shaded land with clucking chickens and scattered fruit trees. Two looms—one empty and another stretching a half-woven rug—stand at the entrance, a ubiquitous sight in Teotitlán. Passing the looms, Beatrice reenters her home to begin cooking breakfast while Alberto goes to help his mother bathe and dress for the day. When Cecilia leaves, Alberto and Beatrice serve breakfast to Juana, who is now sitting in a wheelchair at the dining room table.

Later that day, I met with Cecilia and her family as they recounted the morning's events and reflected on their joint efforts caring for their mother, Juana, an elder in her mid-70s who has grown increasingly dependent. Juana's husband died of diabetes five years ago and, since then, her own health has declined. She has become increasingly forgetful and needs reminding when family members like Cecilia leave home. Yet their most pressing concern is Juana's severe osteoporosis that significantly impacts her mobility. Cecilia and her family reflected on how pitching in and adopting different responsibilities in caring for Juana allows each of them to maintain what they called a "normal life" in the context of their mother's decline. They continue to farm and make money by selling rugs to a local merchant. Cecilia continues to have opportunity to socialize at the market, while Alberto and Beatrice proceed to run other weekly errands in Tlacolula and Oaxaca City. When there are *fiestas*, Cecilia typically remains at home to care for Juana, but for more important family occasions, she and her brother collaborate to transport their mother in a wheelchair.

Juana has difficulty moving through the house, and this is the major challenge facing Cecilia and her family. "What concerns us is her severe osteoporosis," Cecilia said. Juana cannot move without assistance from a wheelchair or walker, and risks falling when she tries to walk across their uneven dirt courtyard. "She always wants to move around," Cecilia continued. "That's what I experience as the hardest part about my experience with her . . . physically helping her get around our house and out of her room." Cecilia described how she, Alberto, and Beatrice also coordinate efforts to cook, bathe, and ensure the safety of their mother so that she does not fall. Juana continues to attempt to participate in household chores like preparing food or washing dishes, but these activities are more to help Juana feel involved in family life than contributions to manage the challenges of everyday life.

It is in the context of these challenges that Cecilia and her family have also noticed Juana become more forgetful. This began shortly after the death of Juana's husband, and the family believed Juana's forgetfulness was an expression of her stress and sadness. Initially, Juana seemed to only forget seemingly trivial things like the comings and goings of Cecilia and family members, but more recently she has begun to forget more significant events. For example, Juana continues to forget that one of her granddaughters has married and relocated to live with her husband's family in another part of town. And similarly, Juana forgets that her other adult son, Pancho, has recently migrated to the United States.

A doctor in Oaxaca City diagnosed Juana with senile dementia four years ago during an osteoporosis consultation, but Cecilia, Alberto, and Beatrice expressed that this didn't concern them or impact their relationship with their mother. As discussed in the previous chapter, the doctor explained the difference between senile dementia and Alzheimer's disease, stating that the former only involves forgetting a limited number of things. "She doesn't completely forget," Beatrice explained, and went on to describe how they are not worried because Juana has not completely lost her ability to remember. "She forgets little things, like if one of us goes out and she then asks where we went, even though we told her earlier where we were going," Beatrice said. "So we thought all of this was normal to us, since everyone forgets things. . . . In fact, her forgetfulness is only temporary since when we remind her where we're going—or where we went—then she says she remembers."

If Juana's forgetfulness—understood to be just little things, and only temporary—was not worrying, I wondered what kind of forgetfulness would be a cause for concern. To find out, I asked Beatrice about the importance of memory. Where she drew the line—between common forgetfulness and a type of memory loss that would be concerning—was centered on ideas about family cohesion. As noted in the previous chapter, Beatrice said that memory is important "because we have kids and I have a husband. I can't even imagine that I could forget that I have children or forget that I have a husband." Beatrice's comments help highlight how she was able to minimize her mother-in-law's forgetfulness and also how "complete forgetting" invokes the inherent segre-social dynamics in caregiving experience. Forgetfulness is not merely a symptom of cognitive decline, but also indexed to the foreclosure of family and social cohesion, values most at stake in Teotitlán today. Indeed, in a setting where cohesion is undermined by broader social change, this perspective highlights how social issues inform even the basic experience and meaning of forgetfulness itself (see also Berkman et al., 2005; Guarnaccia, Good, Good, & Kleinman, 1990; Guarnaccia et al., 1992).

Central to making sense of this observation is the anthropological concept of idioms of distress, defined as "socially and culturally resonant means of experiencing and expressing distress in local worlds" (Nichter, 2010, p. 405). First pioneered by Mark Nichter (1981), idioms of distress provide an avenue to study how individuals' talk about illness—that is, the idioms they use—is "culturally constituted" and expressive of broader social horizons (p. 379). Beatrice's comment about "complete forgetting" is one example, where her experience of forgetfulness is constituted within a social setting concerned about the maintenance of family cohesion. Yet the original significance of this approach is important because it shifts attention from the *content* of cultural difference (for example, that some cultures talk about Alzheimer's disease whereas others normalize forgetting) toward the pragmatic *function* of those differences (for example, how talk about Alzheimer's serves a specific social purpose). Pragmatism is at the heart of addressing why idioms of distress matter.[1] As Nichter (2010) later reformulates it, inquiring "Why this?" is instrumental toward appreciating how idioms of distress are not just constitutive of—but are pragmatic responses to—cultural surroundings.[2]

From my perspective as a clinical psychologist, asking why caregivers like Cecilia are (not) concerned about forgetfulness is important. It directs attention away from mere facts we have garnered about conditions like Alzheimer's disease as being caused by underlying neurological pathology, toward simultaneously considering the way people variably experience and understand forgetfulness. Moreover, it importantly highlights the pragmatic function that those differences serve in everyday life, in this case, the way that viewing forgetfulness as normal helps foster a certain sense of family cohesion.

Attention to cultural difference and pragmatic function helps contain a tendency in the clinical science that overlooks cultural dimensions of illness. So often, clinicians like myself approach people's varying experiences and understandings of illness from *within* a scientific framework—as either being "correct" in agreeing with what science tells us about the cause of illness or "incorrect" in overlooking those insights. Further, when we encounter cultural variants of illness, we tend to translate those differences into concepts we already understand. It is not difficult to imagine, for example, that the normality Cecilia described in her mother's forgetfulness would be translated as an instance of Alzheimer's disease. But this, in turn, leads us to overlook how different cultural settings varyingly constitute illness. It leads us to overlook how what Cecilia describes of normal forgetfulness represents a truth in itself. This is not just my opinion, but something that is expressed in the *DSM-5* (2013), the diagnostic textbook for mental health professionals. "Cultural concepts of distress," a derivative of Nichter's work, are defined as different experiences, social expressions, and causal understandings of illness. The DSM describes specific examples of cultural concepts and goes on to state, "*all* forms of distress are locally shaped—including DSM disorders" and further specifies "there is seldom a one-to-one correspondence of any cultural concept with a DSM diagnostic entity" (p. 758).

The authors of the *DSM* are certainly on the right track. But in my experience as a clinician, this sensibility continues to be overlooked. A large part of this comes from the truth claims clinicians like myself adopt in understanding illness, involving what Good (1996) terms the "epistemological ambivalence" in assuming that some understandings of illness are more accurate than others.

While clinicians might appreciate that different cultures have different cultural experiences of illness, we continue to translate and reduce those differences into an epistemology (biomedical, cognitive, behavioral, psychoanalytic, and so forth) that we think *more accurately* accounts for phenomena. Progressive forgetfulness might not be alarming to some cultures, for example, but we (clinicians) *know* that it is expressive of underlying neuropathology. Maintaining this stance is sensible in some instances (like in helping families anticipate the future), but it simultaneously overlooks what is distressing to individuals as they encounter illness in the moment. Assuming that one knows more about the reality of another person's experience overlooks key elements of that person's experience. Returning to Nichter's emphasis on the functionality of idioms—asking why and how idioms directly impact life—helps contain this epistemological objection and appreciate cultural variants of illness in their own terms. This is the essence of the type of cultural pragmatism I am defending throughout this book.

In this chapter, I turn to study Cecilia and other caregivers' idioms to account for their experience and understanding of age-related progressive forgetfulness, what would often be labeled Alzheimer's disease in other settings. With specific focus on the symptoms and etiologies of Alzheimer's, I explore how caregivers see and understand progressive forgetfulness and forge meaningful relationships with elders in its context. In general, this chapter aims to show how talk about progressive forgetfulness is at once expressive of concern about social cohesion, while also of caregivers' pragmatic efforts to pursue meaningful lives in this context. In so doing, I simultaneously explore how attending to idioms of distress points toward an alternative epistemology rooted in pragmatism, accounting for the way various *truths* are created and maintained based on their social usefulness.

THE SPECTRUM OF FORGETFULNESS: "COMPLETE" FORGETTING IN THE CONTEXT OF SOCIAL CHANGE

Through the course of my fieldwork I had the opportunity to meet families who cared for elders in different stages of what would be called Alzheimer's disease—a spectrum of progressive memory loss ranging from those elders whose symptoms seemed benign, to a type of forgetfulness that was unquestionably pathological. Alberto, Beatrice, and Cecilia represent a case in the middle. Juana was able to remember key events and family members, but has begun to show difficulty remembering the goings-on of daily life. She needs to be reminded when family members like Cecilia have left home to do errands, but also forgets more serious events like her granddaughter's recent move to live in a different home with her husband. Yet to appreciate this family's under-standing of Juana's forgetfulness—and how they perceive it to be different from "complete forgetting"—it helps to contextualize it with others. The total set of voices I encountered in my research illustrates that forgetfulness is largely experienced in context to a broader concern about family cohesion, and is representative of caregivers' pragmatic attempts to respond to it. This is to say, the way forgetfulness is perceived is shaped by what can be done about it. This draws upon what Charles Goodwin (1994) terms a "practice-based theory of knowledge and action," attending to how the very things people notice and take to be objective is not an act of cognitive transparency of the world, but is rather mediated by broader social activities—"practices"—that implicitly structure vision itself. Indeed, as John Dewey (1925/1998) observed in his writings on pragmatism, "the function of intelligence is . . . not that of copying the objects of the environment, but rather of taking account of the way in which more effective and more profitable relations with these objects may be established in the future" (p. 10). In this way, the following spectrum of how caregivers see forgetfulness is not an unmediated depiction of "objective" symptoms, but an encounter with symptoms in the context of social change.

The most moderate description of forgetfulness I found was in the household of Luis and Laura, a married couple in their mid-40s. They jointly provide care for Laura's mother, a recently widowed elder in her mid-70s who they deemed to need help with managing household affairs. After moving in with her, Luis and Laura began to notice the regularity of forgetfulness. I was particularly struck by their lighthearted tone in describing these instances.

> Luis: She often forgets her bag.
> Laura: [*laughs*] Her money.
> Luis: For example, when she wakes up—when she gets out of her room—she'll get her bag ready and [she'll] leave it at the entrance, and she goes back to her room. And then she starts asking where her bag is. And that kind of surprises us, because it happens so often.

The levity of this exchange is perhaps best explained by Luis and Laura's lack of concern. Laura laughs at her husband's observation, and then supplements it with her own. Here, forgetting appears benign, ordinary, a simple instance of inattentiveness that I suspect most readers can relate to. The forgetfulness in Laura's mother poses no major hindrance to family functioning and can easily be overlooked. But Luis also curiously says that the elder's forgetfulness nevertheless strikes him as strange. He is surprised about the frequency with which his mother-in-law forgets, the number of times she is confused about where her belongings are. Indeed, I came to meet with this family because Luis and Laura had told people about their experience (who then relayed their stories to me)—further indicating that they found this behavior "surprising." In this way, minor forgetfulness is something caregivers are aware of, but is nevertheless a condition they minimize.

This exchange helps provide greater context to the perspective about "complete forgetting" that was used to differentiate the symptoms observed by Cecilia and her family. Every morning when Cecilia leaves home, she tells her mother that she is going to the market and will be back shortly but, not long after, Juana asks about where Cecilia has gone. Indeed, this was one of the dominant symptoms noted by Cecilia's family to indicate that Juana has begun to forget more. But similar to Luis and Laura, forgetfulness is something they also minimize. At one point, Alberto said:

> When she forgets, we don't pay much attention to it, and we feel it's normal because when we get together again, she gets back to normal. But when [my sister] Cecilia goes away, even if she is only doing chores, she always is asking, "Where did she go?" even though she was told where Cecilia went. . . . But, but—to truly forget—she doesn't really forget.

This was another instance where Alberto, Cecilia, and Beatrice expressed aware-ness of their mother's forgetfulness, but minimized it through comparison to a more severe "true" or "complete" form. Despite its regularity, they said that it is not something that significantly impacts or concerns their lives. But in this case, forgetfulness is more severe than the typical misplacement of objects. Juana has difficulty recalling events that structure daily activities. She asks where people like Cecilia have gone, when she was told just moments before. But she also forgets major events like her granddaughter's marriage. All these signify that Juana's experience of the world has become more disintegrated. And yet, like Luis and Laura, Alberto continues to minimize the importance of his mother's forgetfulness. He minimizes it by observing that she can remember at other times, and says that she appears to return to "normal" when the family has reunited. Juana's apparent return to normalcy lends additional perspective regarding how forgetfulness is indexed to concern about social cohesion. For-getfulness is understood to manifest in the context of instances when the family is rendered apart, and is something that can be ameliorated when the family has reunited. This ability to return to normal is what differentiates the type of forgetfulness these caregivers witness in daily life, compared to the type of complete or total forgetting that they view as more serious.

Differentiating between "complete" and "normal" forms of forgetting occurred even among caregivers who dealt with more concerning symptoms. Sergio's family (featured in chapter 1) discussed how they were often aware of Pedro's forgetfulness and understood it to be connected to his dangerous tendency to wander, like when he got lost in Tijuana. Nevertheless, they said that Pedro's forgetfulness is something they tend to laugh off and view without concern.

> SERGIO: One time I was coming back home and he [my father] asked me, "Who's your dad?" [*Family laughs in unison.*]
>
> LINDA: Oh, last year one of my daughters came back home, and when she arrived to the house she was very happy. And then my husband asked her, "Who are you?" And my daughter told him, "I'm your daughter." And he said that he didn't believe her, and he laughed. So he forgets. Even now he confuses his children. He will switch their names and he would call Sergio "Manuel," and Manuel "Sergio." And he always confuses them.

For Sergio and family, forgetfulness means more than just misplacing objects or forgetting ordinary events. It involves difficulty remembering basic information and remaining safe. Family members are forgotten, public streets are a liability to become lost in, and in general there is a more serious threat to Pedro's sense of coherence in the world. Yet what is interesting is not that memory problems can become more severe, but rather that Sergio's family response is so similar to other caregivers despite them encountering a more severe instance of forgetfulness. They continue to laugh. They minimize Pedro's forgetfulness even when his safety appears jeopardized and he has greater difficulty remembering the family.

In fact, nearly all caregiving households who dealt with cases of progressive forgetfulness talked about how they were aware of elders' symptoms while saying it is something they overlook and consider to be normal. More than this, they laugh. The anthropologist Michael Jackson (2017) writes that "laughter springs from an ambiguous situation" of interpersonal relating where contradictory understandings or perspectives collide (pp. 137–144). Here, laughter is expressive of the juxtaposition between elders as they have historically been known as figures of authority, and now as persons who display symptoms of forgetfulness.

Elders' forgetfulness stands in contrast to their authority. So, caregivers laugh. Yet another way to account for this behavior is through the nature of language itself, and the way in which talk about forgetfulness shapes caregivers' experience of it. Semioticians influenced by pragmatism (for example, Morris, 1971) and social scientists influenced by Michel Foucault (for example, Packer, 2010; Potter, 2003; Kendall & Wickham, 1998) point to how language has constitutive power in the social world. Each of these researchers is at least implicitly influenced by Austin's (1975) perspective that language does not merely describe, but has performative functions—it *does* things—and these functions have concrete effects on the surrounding world (see also Laugier, 2013, pp. 97–109). Caregivers' talk about forgetfulness as something that is normal changes their worldview; it constructs a perspective that at once acknowledges symptoms while simultaneously minimizing their importance.

Although appealing to the nature of language helps explain how caregivers are able to experience forgetfulness as normal, it does not address Nichter's pragmatic question about *why* they do it. And merely observing that something is a function of language does not go far enough to explain the reason speech manifests this way. This question is especially pertinent to readers in the United States, where age-related forgetfulness is noted with such hyperacuity and alarm (Ballenger, 2006; Post, 2000). But in contrast to this outlook, Teotitecos' view of forgetfulness makes sense in context and in general. In the most general sense and likely across most cultural settings, a major part of social interactions is premised on overlooking peculiarities of another person's speech in order to establish a sense of common understanding. Drawing on pragmatism's emphasis on function, language is designed to foster social interaction. We tend to find meaning in what other people say despite the ambiguity, irrationality, and opaqueness that surround language. That is because, in the words of Donald Davidson (1984), we maintain a "principle of charity," an assumption that other people are rational agents and that it is our responsibility as listener to decipher the meaning they seek to convey.[3]

But that even caregivers who deal with more-severe symptoms of forgetfulness view it to be normal moves this idea beyond a general statement about the nature of language and toward an observation specific to Teotitlán. Why do caregivers like Sergio, Manuel, and Linda state that their father's inability to recall members of the family is normal when it so clearly is a divergence from prior life experiences? Perhaps the most convincing answer is through taking on Arthur Kleinman's (1997) emphasis on what is "at stake" if they risk claiming that forgetfulness is not normal. At stake is not only caregivers' ability to form meaningful relations with elders, but also how their relationships symbolize a broader sense of cohesion within the family and community. Similar to Lawrence Cohen's (1998) observation about how elders with dementia in India were perceived to have a "hot voice" that suggested they lived in a "bad family" that failed to uphold normative expectations, instances of forgetfulness in Teotitlán also carry broader social meanings. Both among caregivers in the home and their imagination of being perceived by neighbors in the community, the presence forgetful elders highlight how family and social cohesion—as well as local norms about caregiving for elders—are now viewed to be endangered. This concerns how the community engages and responds to influences perceived to be foreign, as members of households migrate to pursue economic opportunities away, and as broader globalizing trends are introduced back home.

In this context, caregivers' statements about forgetfulness being normal are efforts to bolster what every Teotiteco implicitly views to be endangered, the integrity of the family unit and, by extension, cohesion within the larger community. Talk about forgetfulness as normal promotes certain ideals centering on social cohesion in the context of "modern" social change that is perceived to undermine those ideals (see also Ochs & Kremer-Sadlik, 2015). That is why, in line with the pragmatists, viewing forgetfulness as normal does not derive from some abstract local notion of normalness, but rather something Teotitecos *want* affirmed. Pragmatism is so relevant to account for caregivers' experience and talk about forgetfulness because it puts into focus how perspectives of illness occur within larger concerns about what illness is perceived to threaten. As James (1907/2000) writes about the way we hold certain things to be true, "The really vital question for us all is, What is this world going to be?" (p. 57). This question stands not only at the heart of how individuals make sense of the world, but to their very perception of what the world looks like. James's question captures the ways pragmatic sensibilities shape the nature of experience itself. In the case of the caregivers discussed above, taking on this question highlights how forgetfulness is viewed in regard to the importance of social cohesion.

Though this observation appeared valid throughout my fieldwork, I found certain exceptions in more-severe cases. These approximated descriptions of what Cecilia and other caregivers understood as "complete" or total memory loss associated with Alzheimer's disease. Here, instead of using the Zapotec word for the forgetfulness of objects (*rienlá'az*), these descriptions now centered on the word for forgetfulness of people (*raguenlá'az*). For example, Carlos, an elder in his midseventies, described his experience of jointly providing care with his adult children for his wife, Cynthia. Six years ago, Cynthia began exhibiting symptoms similar to the ones described above—forgetting daily happenings like family members temporarily leaving home (information conveyed to her moments prior)—but then more regularly forgetting important recent events. Now, Cynthia's forgetfulness has progressed such that she is unable to recognize members of the family who reside at home, and she has difficulty maintaining a basic conversation. She was diagnosed with Alzheimer's and, since then, Carlos and his family described how they have become responsible for more-intimate dimensions of his wife's well-being, such as feeding and bathing her, as well as assisting her in the bathroom. Despite Carlos's family's efforts to integrate her into the household, they described how his wife was now unable to appropriately respond and maintain a sense of understanding of the world around her. At one point, Carlos stated that he cannot pretend his relationship is normal because Cynthia's memory has become "completely lost." Carlos further elaborated: "She doesn't remember anything anymore. And if you talk to her she won't listen. And even if she listens she won't answer... And when she answers she answers completely off topic. That's how I realize that she's not aware anymore. You can't hold a conversation with her." In describing this experience and the progress of decline they've witnessed over the years, Carlos and his family did not laugh or attempt to normalize Cynthia's forgetfulness. His use of the word "completely" points to how Cynthia not only fails to recollect information, but how she is no longer able to uphold a semblance of familial cohesion. She does not recognize members of the family or recall distant memories, and her basic speech is compromised. Both the charity and the pragmatic function of language observed in other caregiving households were no longer tenable. Through this instance of more-severe forgetting, we gain insight into the concrete limitations of how forgetfulness is pragmatically normalized.

Taken as a whole, each of the caregivers featured above illustrates a moment along the spectrum of progressive forgetfulness. On one hand, this spectrum is congruent with how Alzheimer's disease is classified according to early, mid-, and late-stage symptoms in the United States and other biomedically oriented settings. In Teotitlán as elsewhere, these forms of forgetfulness are progressive: memory problems become more noticeable and problematic with time. Yet this spectrum also highlights specific ways age-related progressive forgetfulness is perceived locally, and how differentiating between "normal" and "complete" forms of forgetfulness pragmatically serves specific social functions. Up to a critical point, the very symptoms that caregivers notice of forgetful elders are shaped by concern for social cohesion; caregivers continually overlook and minimize those symptoms while emphasizing evidence that their relationships feel cohesive and their households remain functioning. In this way, caregivers' perceptions of forgetfulness are not objective readings of external events but interpretations of those events in the context of their desires about how they want to live.

ETIOLOGICAL UNDERSTANDINGS: CAREGIVERS BECOME AGENTS OF ACTION

Appreciating how Cecilia, Alberto, and Beatrice differentiated between types of forgetfulness was also relevant for when they discussed their uncle, Manny, an elder they curiously described as being "completely forgetful." They referenced Uncle Manny throughout and often used descriptions of his behavior to minimize what they observed of Juana. Prior to his death ten years ago and before Juana grew forgetful herself, Manny was known for his high temper and poor impulse control. He came to regularly enter Cecilia's home uninvited and unannounced, and walked to the kitchen to eat uncooked and unsanitary foods. He had major difficulty sustaining conversation and often grew irritable and aggressive when people tried to reason with him. And he showed no indication that he remembered anyone's name or relation in the family. "He was really nuts," Beatrice reflected, explaining how this sort of behavior contrasted to the gregarious and respectable person Manny was known to be in earlier years, before his forgetfulness progressed. Yet despite being labeled as completely forgetful, and even being diagnosed by a physician who said that he had Alzheimer's disease, Manny's family viewed his decline through local notions about soul loss. "When the doctor said he had [Alzheimer's] disease, our relatives did not believe it; they thought he was lying," Beatrice said.

Through reflecting on the debated cause for Manny's behavior, I came to appreciate how local views of forgetfulness are not only indexed to concerns about social change, but also are varyingly interpreted via different, plural medical systems.[4] Beatrice's perspective of her family's belief and their disagreement with the doctor's explanation is a larger example of how two medical systems coexist and the power dynamics inherent to this situation.[5]

Like most rural Mexican communities, Teotitlán is situated within a traditional medical system (a system that is itself a syncretic combination of various medical theories from multiple points in history) and a biomedical one (an increasingly dominant perspective about health and illness associated locally with social modernization).[6] Any visitor to Teotitlán can readily detect biomedicine's influence: the government-sponsored health clinic is on the main road that leads to Teotitlán and is visited by neighboring communities who choose not to travel to Oaxaca City for treatment. And, in addition to the allopathic doctors at this clinic, there are other community doctors in private practice, as well as regular publicly sponsored healthcare events put on by Mexico's pension systems (Prospera for the adult population and 70 y Más for elders), such that biomedicine strongly influences local understanding and treatment of illness.

Alongside this system exists traditional medicine, another option that was often mentioned whenever illness was discussed. Yet what so many participants would refer to when they spoke of "traditional medicine" does not originate from undiluted indigenous custom, but rather from a fusion of indigenous ideas with those introduced by the Spanish. This history is complicated but merits attention given how prominent medical ideas appear throughout the pages of this book.[7] Prior to the arrival of the Spaniards who conquered Oaxaca in 1521, the Zapotec understanding of human nature was based within a larger cosmological order that incorporated ideas of equilibrium, psychosocial development, and divine rule.[8] With regard to health beliefs, we know in general that Mesoamerican metaphysics did not distinguish between mind and body, and so understandings of health were based on ecological harmony, and illness was viewed as a divine consequence of social transgression (Rubel, 1960; Somolinos d'Ardois, 1973).[9] Adding to this perspective, the Spanish arrival to Mexico introduced new ideas about medicine and illness via two main conduits. First, the Spanish created a formal network of hospitals and a medical board to issue licenses to doctors and pharmacists. This formal network helped ensure practitioners properly adhered to Greek-based humoral theory, the dominant medical theory that viewed health as constituted by the balance of certain humors ("fluids") and illness as respective imbalance (Hernández Sáenz & Foster, 2001, p. 22).[10] Second, medical ideas were also transmitted informally via *medicinas caseras* (home remedies) brought by the Conquistadores, who had their own folk conceptions of illness and medicine (Hernández Sáenz & Foster, 2001, p. 23). Folk illnesses like *mal de ojo* (evil eye), *susto* (fright), *pérdida del alma* (soul loss)—medical conditions that I found participants describing as "traditional"—were introduced through this second conduit. Yet despite efforts to first displace indigenous medicine and later replace folk theories, the Spanish never totally succeeded. Medical ideas were rather synthesized in a process of acculturation, an ongoing evolution and eventual fusion with multiple systems of medicine (Beltrán, 1992). The "traditional" medicine that exists today in Oaxaca is a product of this complicated history. Contemporary traditional healers recognize illness categories like *pérdida del alma* (folk ideas introduced informally), understand illness as being a result of physical and mental imbalances (humoral theory introduced formally), and offer treatment through administering local herbs and other techniques (drawn from indigenous medical knowledge).

In the following pages I present caregivers' varying understandings for why elders progressively forget. Similar to the syncretic history that marks traditional medicine, each etiology is not based within a discrete medical theory, but rather draws on multiple theories from biomedical and traditional medical systems, illustrating the complex, regenerative ways caregivers are simultaneously situated in a globalizing world and responsive to change within it. As Kaja Finkler (2001) writes of her own study in Mexico, "to know the cause of a sickness is to make sense of one's suffering. . . . [Etiologies] furnish a window to people's ideologies, morality, social interaction, and relations to themselves, their bodies, and their environment" (p. 31). The etiological understandings noted among caregivers provide a similar prism onto their lives. They provide perspective on ways that local notions of forgetfulness are indexed to views about stress and associated social change.

Indeed, given how the previous chapter describes the way age-related forgetfulness is so commonly indexed to stress, what follows is an account of the various etiologies caregivers employ to explain stress and how they view stress as causing progressive forgetfulness. Informed by the influential descriptions of stress pioneered in the work of Hans Selye (1956), most readers take it as a given that the experience of stress leads to physiological and psychological illness. This Euro-American idea also circulates in Oaxaca, as indicated by the fact that Alzheimer's disease is widely held by locals not to exist because of the purported *absence* of modern stress associated with capitalistic lifestyles. In Teotitlán, the Zapotec expression associated with stress—*rak garlien*—points to the distress a person endures, which literally describes "a distressed heart." But Zapotec also has other ways to describe stress, and each has a connotation that points toward perceptions of modern, capitalistic lifestyles. The expression *trabajru ridedu lua* refers to circumstances that demand a lot of work or effort (implying an association to industrial labor). And further, the Zapotec expression *raka estresar* (I am stressed) is also regularly used but, as another illustration of the association of stress to modern life, it is a relatively new expression and draws on the Spanish cognate *estrés* (stress). In each of these expressions, stress is viewed as a causal antecedent to physical and mental ailments and a "modern" experience that is indexed to capitalistic lifestyles (see also Berkman et al., 2005).

Once again, the point in describing these etiologies is to further demonstrate how syncretic health understandings are pragmatic in nature. They are not based on caregivers' stances about what is "objectively" occurring to account for forgetfulness, but are rather oriented toward pragmatically responding to challenges inherent to caregivers' experience of it. This involves what Dewey (1925/1998) terms pragmatism's "metaphysical implication" (p. 8)—that is, how what we take to be true involves a temporal horizon that not only considers information gathered from the past, but also includes possibilities for the future (see also Pierce, 1905, p. 173). The following etiologies are not mere explanations about forgetfulness; they are statements and social projects to build a better future in the context of it. They show how understandings about the cause of illness open a space for caregivers to become agents of action to pragmatically do something in response to the conditions they face.

Soul Loss and Fright: "He forgot where he put his donkey"

A common way to explain forgetfulness was through notions about soul loss and fright.[11] When discussing what they knew of Uncle Manny, Alberto, Beatrice, and Cecilia said that the doctor's diagnosis was contested via local knowledge about soul loss. This discussion came up after they were asked whether the doctor could have helped Manny:

> BEATRICE: I don't know . . . because he [Manny] did go to the doctor once and when the doctor said he had that [Alzheimer's] disease, our relatives did not believe it; they thought he was lying. And they [the family] believed this happened to him because once he went to the mountains and he fell asleep there, that's what they said, right? That's why that happened.
> ALBERTO [interrupts]: *Bianan* [soul loss; Spanish: *pérdida del alma*], he forgot where he put his donkey.

In Teotitlán bianan occurs when an individual is abruptly taken away from a place—or experiences a shock or trauma—and subsequently becomes irritable. Typically associated with vulnerable individuals (children and older adults), the affected person is said to have lost his or her soul.[12] It is a condition where the person is physically alive but, in some subtle way, is different and no longer him- or herself. In the story told by Alberto and his family, Uncle Manny was in the field letting his livestock graze and, after being shocked from an unknown cause, forgets where he put his donkey. He returns home and is perceived by his family to be impatient, forgetful, and no longer the same person.

A related illness category, xhibi (fright or fear; Spanish: susto), was similarly employed to make sense of forgetfulness. The idea behind susto is that a sudden shock or traumatic event causes part of the self to leave the body. Susto has been researched in Teotitlán (Fitzsimmons, 1972) and is more widely recognized as an illness category across Latino cultures (APA, 2013; Rubel, 1960). Locally, susto and soul loss are treated as two separate illness categories, but they are conceptually related. Susto (a shock) is understood to be one of the causes of soul loss—though not all cases of susto lead to soul loss, and there are also other circumstances (like spirit intrusion) where a person may lose his or her soul.

Speculation about susto came up when Linda, Sergio, and Manuel (discussed in chapter 1) reflected on Pedro's past, and considered how frightening events might have caused his forgetfulness today. At one point Linda said:

> Yes, there was this thing that happened to him when he was younger. Because they used to have cattle in the mountains. So he went by himself to herd the cattle. And he realized there were two dogs chasing him. Then, as he was running, he entered into an unknown place. It looked to him as if he was running through mud. He made it running through the mud, but then he got stuck. So he stopped and started walking back. And then he saw an enormous person. And then he realized it was the devil. It had horns. And then he got scared and didn't know how to escape.

This exchange provides insight into how past incidents of susto are used to explain forgetfulness in the present. Linda recalls an event she knows happened to her husband decades ago. She cites this incident to speculate on a possible cause of her husband's current forgetfulness, implying that these past injuries may have resurfaced to cause her husband to forget. This makes sense, given how she believes her husband suffered from forgetfulness immediately after experiencing susto. But Linda later states that she does not know if this explanation is valid. After introducing the idea, her son, Sergio, contests it, while Manuel says he is undecided. Though Linda's suggestion is left as a tentative hypothesis, it nevertheless illustrates the broader point that ideas about susto are locally accepted reasons to explain age-related forgetfulness.

These understandings illustrate how etiologies are functionally communicative in the sense Nichter originally outlined: expressive of modern, social parameters that open up a pragmatic space for action. As Carlos said when he first learned that his wife had Alzheimer's disease: "Well, we [initially] just let it go because we thought there could be a cure for it. But then [the doctor] said that there was no cure." As in other rural Oaxacan settings, of the caregivers whose elders were diagnosed as having Alzheimer's, they were also told that there was little to be done to reverse, arrest, or mitigate disease progress. There is no local arena to deal with Alzheimer's. As will be further discussed in chapter 5, in the entire state of Oaxaca there exist three nursing homes, few geriatric specialists, and few pharmaceutical options. Each of these spheres has very little to do with the treatment of Alzheimer's. Hence, and in contrast to the options to do something about Alzheimer's in U.S. settings, in Oaxaca the same diagnosis is paired with limited relevant choices and forecloses meaningful ways for families to respond. Belief in soul loss thus opens up a new possibility to do something, to seek medical treatment from local healers and engage with the community by adhering to local medical tradition.[13] This is the spirit of pragmatism as James (1907/2000) describes it: "the attitude of looking away from first things, principles, 'categories,' supposed necessities; and of looking towards last things, fruits, consequences, and facts" (p. 29). Etiologies are furnished not in reference to some abstract, underlying idea of cause, not deduced from an abstract understanding of biomedicine or other medical frameworks. Rather, those frameworks are appealed to *because* caregivers intuit that they might have a function—in this case, belief in soul loss furnishes hope for other medical systems to respond to the symptoms that cannot be treated by current biomedical options.

Thinking Too Much and Sadness: "Thinking from the heart"

This pragmatic sensibility can equally be detected in caregivers' views about sadness and related ruminative symptoms. Indeed, "thinking too much" has been a widely studied construct across cultural groups and appears as a cultural concept of distress in the *DSM-5* (APA, 2013, p. 858; Kaiser et al., 2015). Mexican immigrants in the United States commonly cite thinking too much as a symptom of depression associated with migration and nostalgia for home communities (Martinez Tyson et al., 2011) and, inversely, in a similar Nicaraguan setting, grandmother caregivers who remain at home have been known to experience it in relation to the challenges associated in caring for grandchildren left by mothers who have migrated abroad (Yarris, 2014, 2017). Similarly in Teotitlán, the Zapotec word to refer to sadness, *naban*, is used as a conditional state of being in sentences like *naban yuan*, meaning, "S/he is sad." Once more, caregivers not only used this general condition as a symptom to describe forgetfulness, but also as an etiology that opened functional possibilities in its context.

Carlos, the husband who cared for his "completely lost" wife with severe Alzheimer's, provides one example of how sadness is mobilized to explain forgetfulness.[14] Although Carlos was a well-regarded lawyer in the community, he and his family continued to also be known for weaving high-end rugs. When she was healthy, Carlos and his wife wove to continue the family legacy, but also as a means to spend time among each other and with their adult children. Like the majority of Teotitecos, they viewed this work as a major facet of their social identities. Yet Cynthia had lived with diabetes for the majority of her adult life and, ten years ago, she had a finger amputated because of it. "She liked to work a lot, and when this [amputation] happened, she considered herself useless," explained her adult son, Francisco. Carlos elaborated further:

> Well, since she's diabetic, what we think caused [her forgetfulness]. . . .
> She had one of her fingers amputated. . . . It got infected so it had
> to be amputated. That's when she started to ruminate [Zapotec
> original: *rikiela'z*; literally: "to think a lot from the heart"]. That's what
> we think caused [her forgetfulness]. That's why it started gradually.
> She couldn't handle all that thinking.

Her being debilitated, Carlos speculated that Cynthia lost her social identity, leading to her feeling alienated from family and the larger community. This caused her to withdraw, think too much, and ultimately become forgetful.[15] Her thinking from the heart was a symptom of the gradual foreclosure of her social identity. Such an explanation was an important attempt for Carlos and his family to empathize and understand his wife's forgetfulness as an underlying expression of her social pain. Forgetfulness again is indexed to a condition that caregivers can attempt to engage with and respond to. To further this last point, Sophia, another caregiver, described how her forgetful husband thought a lot from the heart and, in her descriptions, came to account for how her husband was nostalgic (Zapotec original: *ragwenlaz*; literally "a clenched heart") and full of sadness (Zapotec original: *riberuu*). These accounts are not just descriptions of forgetfulness, but attempts to pragmatically respond to its underlying cause.

Caregivers were not the only ones who appealed to this etiology. They also noted how elders themselves cited thinking too much as a way to understand their own forgetfulness. This was most salient during an interview with Pablo and Vanessa, a married couple who reflected on their experience caregiving for an elder diagnosed with Alzheimer's disease. Yet in comparison to how Carlos and his family used sadness to understand Cynthia's forgetfulness, here Pablo and Vanessa say that the elder herself appeals to her own ruminative sadness to explain why she has become forgetful.

> VANESSA: When I talk to her I ask why she forgets. . . . Well, what she says is that it is probably because she thinks about a lot of things that happened throughout her life. What happened to them [the elder and her deceased husband] when they lived here [in Teotitlán]. And that's what has affected her the most. A lot of thinking. That's when she says that she forgets.
>
> PABLO: And also because her husband passed away, and he was buried there [in Mexico City]—they weren't able to bring him back, because they weren't able to pay the expenses to have the funeral in town. That's what affected her the most . . .
>
> VANESSA: There was a time when she would cry in her room, she would even scream. And that's something that also affected her.

This excerpt reads remarkably similar to observations made about Carlos, only here it is the elder who is making her sadness known. The elder in this household left her community to migrate to Mexico City, only to return to Teotitlán lonely as a widow. Despite having returned, she still is impacted by her earlier decision to migrate. Years of living away now make her feel isolated, with few family members to call on. She feels removed from the larger community. The elder's explanation of thinking too much helps Pablo and Vanessa better relate to the elder, and subsequently provides a relevant way to respond to the perceived cause of her forgetfulness.

Appealing to thinking too much and sadness as a cause of forgetfulness shows how adverse life circumstances—what Finkler (2001) calls "life's lesions"— become inscribed on the body and expressed through illness. Focusing on these circumstances helps caregivers make sense of elders' symptoms, attributing the cause of forgetfulness to something they can understand. But it also furnishes a pragmatic response—a means to engage—between caregivers and forgetful elders. In both examples, we see how understanding forgetfulness through this perspective establishes a common understanding and, more importantly, a means of social engagement. In this way, Teotitecos' experiences of sadness and thinking too much were not only expressive of a broader social setting where notions of family and social unity were perceived to be threatened, but also how this very understanding allows for those threats to be challenged.

Forgetfulness as Standard Aging: The Dried-Up Brain

As a final etiological understanding, I now turn to aging as an explanation itself.[16] Many caregivers explained forgetfulness via aging, citing the lifecycle as a sufficient reason for why elders are known to forget.[17] This further explains how caregivers view forgetfulness as normal and nonproblematic. As an etiological understanding, viewing age as the cause of forgetfulness implicitly posits that it is normal to forget and that, as persons age, they tend to exhibit these symptoms more (see also Berkman et al., 2005). This understanding serves to avoid and negate the possible stress that might otherwise account for an elder's forgetfulness.

In light of how forgetfulness tends to be minimized and seen as normal, most caregivers endorsed this view. As an example, I return to my meeting with Sergio, Manuel, and Linda, the caregivers discussed in chapter 1. While they considered susto as being a cause of forgetfulness, they simultaneously questioned whether Pedro was even ill, and instead whether his forgetfulness might owe to normal aging. They reflected on how Pedro has come to progressively show more serious signs of forgetting. "I guess it's gradual," Manuel said, "because as he gets older I believe he's forgetting more." Manuel discussed how Pedro's forgetfulness also arose in conjunction with greater physical limitations, such as knee pain he suffered from working in the fields throughout his life. Because of the way they continued to reference the fact that Pedro was aging, I questioned whether this family understood Pedro's forgetfulness as an illness or something to be expected. Manuel responded: "It could be due to a sort of illness, or it could also be due to his age. That's what I think; it might be because of his age." Manuel entertains the idea that his father's forgetfulness is an illness, but he then concludes that a better interpretation is that age is the cause. Manuel's hesitancy—his willingness to consider this question, but then conclude that forgetfulness "might be" attributable to aging—is also telling. Though he has an intuition about the cause of his father's condition, he concludes that he ultimately does not know. This illustrates how etiological understandings are tentatively held, and sheds better insight onto the way caregivers like Manuel hold multiple ideas about illness at the same time.[18]

Understanding forgetfulness as being caused by aging presupposes certain ideas about the aging process in general. Like how Sergio, Manuel, and Linda considered forgetfulness as being related to Pedro's old age, other families endorsed a perspective of aging that hinted at views about how aging occurs, and why aging involves greater cognitive and physical limitations. For example, although Luis and Laura continued to express that the moderate forgetfulness they observed of Laura's mother was not concerning, they also speculated about how age itself was an explanation for her change in behavior. At one point, Luis shared how he views forgetfulness to be a natural part of aging, and then, as if on second thought, explained why he understands forgetfulness to naturally occur. "Most elders forget things due to their old age," Luis said, normalizing the symptoms he noticed in his mother-in-law. "And I think that's because they've used a lot of their brain." Like so many other caregivers, Luis observes that most elders seem to forget things, so he concludes that forgetfulness is a natural part of aging. Yet in the process, Luis makes an important observation about how elders are known to "use up their brain." Here, Luis seems to be implicitly positing a hypothesis that individuals are endowed with a limited amount of resources, and that aging represents the progressive depletion of them. This invokes a common perspective in Oaxaca about the lifecycle as a continual process of desiccation; individuals are born with a certain amount of wet attributes that eventually become used and dried (Royce, 2011, pp. 12–14).[19] In this regard, forgetfulness is understood as a symptom of cognitive depletion, of one's wet, life-sustaining resources turning dry.

Once more, this perspective about the cause of forgetfulness also discloses a realm of action for caregivers to take. Beyond serving to avoid acknowledging stress in elders' lives, this perspective leads to greater empathy and patience about the disruptions that elders' forgetfulness causes. It also fosters understanding among caregivers that they, too, will grow old and may become forgetful. This normalizes age-related forgetfulness by observing that it is a condition every person is liable to develop. In so doing, this etiology again fosters greater interpersonal cohesion and demonstrates how etiological understandings involve more than theoretical explanations of illness, but pragmatic avenues to live with and respond to it.

～

Attending to perceptions and etiological explanations of forgetfulness helps put into focus the cultural pragmatism needed to appreciate people's everyday lived experience, how talk about illness performs culturally specific functions.

The caregivers in this chapter show how idioms of distress go beyond being constructed within social parameters, but are also constructive of the world they want to live in. Congruent with Nichter's original formulation, this chapter has approached idioms of distress by studying not just their perceptible "whatness" (that is, cultural differences) but also by pragmatically asking "why this" (that is, cultural functions). What is noticed of forgetfulness and how it is understood to arise are perspectives that are not merely constituted within and expressive of cultural parameters, but also dynamically responsive to them. This is the larger significance when Nichter suggests researchers and clinicians question *why* people express distress in a particular way, reminding us of the inherent agency of individuals as they encounter, respond, and attempt to ameliorate distress surrounding illness.

By shifting focus from thinking of truth as something that corresponds to an abstract verifiable object toward seeing it as one created based on usefulness, philosophical pragmatism attends to the functionality of idioms of distress without being sidetracked about whether some understandings of illness are more valid than others. According to pragmatists, claims about the causes of illness are valid insofar as they are useful. This approach helps us appreciate cultural differences noted in the symptoms and understandings about the cause of forgetfulness in their own right, and allows us to remain attuned to how those differences represent important strategies to live in the context of illness. Pragmatism at once helps us appreciate the way idioms of distress are constituted within cultural parameters and, more important to the points made in this chapter, are expressive of human agency within them.

As a whole, attending to the pragmatic function of symptoms and etiologies moves beyond studying idioms of distress merely as cultural variants. Rather, attending to these dimensions of illness helps us appreciate how individuals see and make sense of their world based on desired action. As Dewey's (1925/1998) point on metaphysics shows, the whole purpose of thinking is not to make sense of the world in an abstract sense, but to change it. In Teotitlán, caregivers' perceptions and understandings of age-related forgetfulness help enact change by bringing family members together, and also by serving as a means to continue engaging with elders in locally resonant ways. From my stance as a psychologist, these perspectives seem equally as important as neurological ones; they capture the heart of why age-related forgetfulness is distressing and how individuals attempt to pursue meaningful lives in its context.

Attending to the functional nature of idioms of distress further reveals how caregiving reaffirms and regenerates key values perceived to be endangered in contemporary life. This is a setting where family and social cohesion matter, but are put in tension by rifts in social life marked by migration, pursuits of capital gain, and other "modern" modes of being. Viewing forgetfulness as normal and responding to it with concern for social cohesion clads forgetfulness within a social fabric that not only gives caregivers the chance to meaningfully respond to forgetful elders, but also enables them to come together as the community encounters broader social change. In her study of grandmother caregiving in Nicaragua, Kristin Yarris (2017) argues that the dual familial-social function inherent to caregiving itself involves cultural regeneration. "Despite the social hardships and uncertainties of transnational family life, [caregivers] are actively and affirmatively participating in the re-creation of cultural values for family life through their caregiving" (p. 112). In a similar vein, the perspectives explored by caregivers in Teotitlán—that forgetfulness is viewed in context to "modern" stress, and that this perspective subsequently provides opportunities to pragmatically respond to forgetfulness—show how caregiving households simultaneously affirm and regenerate key values perceived to be endangered in contemporary life.

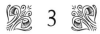

3

Health-Seeking Behavior

POWER AND BELIEF IN MEDICAL DECISION-MAKING

Graciela began to cry when describing the details of her life. At 75 years old, she sat in a child-sized wooden chair that matched her small stature. Her tanned face was wrinkled and her clothes faded of color. At her age it has become difficult to continue earning money by spinning yarn, so she now sells handmade *tortillas* at the local market. Her two adult children are married with their own families and financially contribute less than they once had. And, although she and her husband, Nicholas, each receive a bimonthly pension from 70 y Más, she regularly struggles to earn enough money to buy food and other necessities.[1] "Nowadays, you can't buy much of anything with 20 pesos," she said to reflect on how much more expensive life has become. These troubles have only doubled since her husband's first stroke. "I think what her heart wants is to have him work," explained her son, Mario, upon seeing her cry. Indeed, when I first met her, Graciela was in the middle of hanging threadbare clothes to dry, and we gathered with her family in the shade of their dirt courtyard, enclosed by weathered adobe walls and minimal adornments. There was a notable absence of luxuries like televisions and automobiles I found in other households. And, in general, I had the impression that this family was continually struggling to make ends meet.

Yet for Graciela, these financial hardships were perhaps easier to focus on than others she faced. Since having his first stroke seven years ago, Nicholas has progressively lost functioning and is now completely dependent on family care. He is immobile, gestures to communicate, and needs to be fed. His family cuts his fingernails and shaves his beard, as well as other tasks like helping him eat and using the toilet. "He does it at any time," Mario said, describing his father's incontinence, and then further explained that washing Nicholas's soiled pants has been an ongoing challenge. Mario is also the only member of the household able to physically carry his father from one location to another—to drink *atole* in the kitchen for breakfast, or to get sunshine outside during the afternoons. "But sometimes we see him coming out crawling when we are not there at that moment," Mario said. The family further reflected on how Nicholas's memory has also created hardship. Although they spend most of their time caring for him, Nicholas also shows no indication that he remembers Graciela, their children, or basic facts about the family. "It's difficult," Mario explained, "because you cannot talk to him anymore. You can't talk to him like your dad. He's just become a body."

Mario and his wife, Isabelle, live in the same household as Mario's parents, and together with other family members cobble resources to support Nicholas. They make money by selling rugs to a local merchant, along with a pension and the moderate income made from the tortillas Graciela sells. They are also helped by Fredrico, Mario's brother who had lived in California with his own family for years, but who now has temporarily returned to live in an adjacent home for a two-year *cargo* service. When in California, Fredrico brought clothing, but now that he is in Teotitlán, he comes with his family to help monitor Nicholas. Yet Mario said that he and his mother are the primary persons responsible for Nicholas's care. They assist him to the bathroom, clean his soiled pants, and feed him. "So I think they [Fredrico and his family] have less responsibility," he said. "I always have in mind that I have to monitor him," Mario went on to say. And he further explained how his daily life is nearly entirely structured on providing care to his dependent father, leading to challenges that other family members do not fully recognize.

In contrast to the way progressive forgetfulness was understood by other households in the previous chapter, Graciela's family saw the sudden onset of Nicholas's symptoms in relation to his heavy consumption of alcohol. Nicholas began to drink after the death of his son 20 years ago. "He wouldn't just drink a shot of *mezcal*," Graciela said of Nicholas's history, "he would really drink." And

Isabelle added, "I once saw him [drunk and] crawling just like a baby—I still can't understand why he drank that much." Graciela and her family believe this is what caused the high blood pressure that eventually led to Nicholas's strokes. But although they understood this in context to a biomedical framework of how illness has underlying physiological causes, Graciela and her family also spoke of *susto*, simultaneously invoking traditional understandings. They described the first time Nicholas had a stroke.

> MARIO: What happened is that he got scared when he went to the bathroom.
> ISABELLE: It was in the middle of the night.
> MARIO: "Something appeared," he said. But he didn't tell us what it was. It was shocking for him, because when he left he was fine. But when he returned, he was in a stupor [Zapotec: *kedruzalasdian*, literally, "he doesn't remember"].
> ISABELLE: He then told us that he saw an animal, a very hairy animal, a big animal. [*Isabelle continues in a whisper:*] That's what he thought he saw. And he said that he was very frightened. I don't remember exactly if he said that the animal attacked him, or if it just stood in front of him.
> MARIO: That happened the very first time.
> ISABELLE: That's why we think that that caused what he has now.

As discussed in the previous chapter, susto is a notion of illness that involves a sudden shock that causes part of the self to leave the body. In this episode, susto befell upon Nicholas during an *hora mala* (bad hour), a local perspective that there are specific hours during the night where individuals are vulnerable to spirit intrusion (also known as *mal aire*, or bad air). In Teotitlán and other Mexican settings, it is held that evil spirits might attack during certain hours, and for protection people wear shawls on their head and try to avoid being out during this time (see also Norget, 2006, p. 74). In this way, although Graciela and her family suspect that Nicholas had a predisposition to strokes because of high blood pressure, he went outside to the bathroom during this ominous hour and returned ill.

With the exception of providers who might ally with a particular medical model, rarely are explanatory or treatment models of illness exclusive, and it is the norm across cultures that individuals draw on multiple and overlapping ideas in medically plural landscapes (Good, 2010; Kleinman, 1988a; Leslie, 1980).[2] Though Graciela and her family initially sought help from a *curandera* (traditional healer) to respond to Nicholas's abrupt decline, they also turned to a physician at

Teotitlán's Centro de Salud (local health clinic). "What a doctor relieves is fever and what a curandera relieves is susto. And in this case, both work together. We believe in both of them," Isabelle said to explain her family's engagement with multiple medical systems. Similar to research in other medically plural settings, notions about belief and believing in traditional medicine accounted for this family's turn to a curandera, as well as the broader community's engagement with traditional healers (Pigg, 1996; Young & Garro, 1993). Indeed, there was something inherent about *believing in* medicine that justified its power to heal and be chosen among alternatives.[3]

Central to caregiving in Teotitlán is how medical decisions are made on behalf of another given the plurality of options, invoking what Charles Nuckolls (1991) aptly terms "deciding how to decide," and the way that such decisions involve deeply complicated and overlapping rationales. In this chapter, I address themes in medical anthropology pertaining to health-seeking behavior to explore how caregivers make choices regarding which practitioners to consult and, by extension, which medical systems to engage with (Duncan, 2017b; Ell & Castaneda, 1998; Finkler, 2001b; Kleinman, 1980; Nichter, 1978; Sesia, 1996). In the context of Teotitlán's particular historical and social circumstances, I analyze how caregivers' health-seeking decisions are rooted in epistemological assumptions—beliefs—and how what is held to be true is structured by broader social, political, and economic factors. This is to say, caregivers' medical decisions are not just based on choosing among different medical options about what is held to be most effective, but also on how those options are representative of broader social issues at stake in the community. Caregivers health-seeking behaviors are thus pragmatic responses to these social parameters. This shows how decisions to engage with medical providers represent an additional dimension to the segre-social dynamics inherent in local caregiving experience. Congruent with Rabinow's (1996) point about biosociality that novel biomedical ideas are as likely to produce new modes of identity as they are to reinforce older cultural categories (see also Gibbon & Novas, 2008, p. 6), caregivers are at once caught between alternative perspectives of "tradition" and "modernity": either affirming (and regenerating) idealized notions of what tradition means in contemporary life, or embracing notions of modernity via engagement with biomedicine. Moreover, in making these decisions, caregivers are situated in a tension of being perceived as socially backward or jettisoning local identity, and subject to concomitant stigma in either choice. In this way, this chapter is intended to complement, complicate, and limit the argument I previously made. Whereas in the last chapter I argued that caregivers' understandings of forgetfulness are pragmatic responses that open up alternatives for action, in this chapter I argue that this alone is insufficient to appreciate how caregivers are constituted as health-seeking subjects in Teotitlán. Before, I showed how caregivers endorse multiple etiologies that transcend epistemological perspectives of illness, but here I show how caregivers' decisions about whom to (not) consult invoke other factors that go beyond their relationships with elders, and concern socioeconomic realms of power, as well as broader ideals concerning local tradition and its role in the contemporary world.

TRADITIONAL MEDICAL OPTIONS:
"JUST LIKE OUR ANCESTORS USED TO WORK"

When Graciela saw her husband immediately after his first stroke, she woke from her sleep to find Nicholas holding his pants and wearing his sweater inside-out. He was unable to speak or respond to her questions, and he stood absently staring in the distance. Graciela explained how she was frightened and wanted to find help, but was also worried that doing so would put others in jeopardy during the hora mala. Eventually, she turned to her son, Fredrico, who at that time was visiting from California.

> I went to Fredrico and told him that there's something wrong with his dad. And he asked me, "What's wrong?" And I told him that he just stares in one place, and I don't know what's happening. And he came running—holding a bag of eggs, about four of them. . . . And I told him, "I don't know what's wrong with that man. I didn't see when he went to the bathroom." . . . And so [Fredrico] rubbed the eggs on him, over his entire body. And he said, "We're going to take these [eggs] to the curandera." It was around 4:00 in the morning. . . . So [Fredrico and Mario] went. They immediately went, so she could tell us what's wrong with him. Moments later, they returned and said it was the hora mala. He inhaled the air of the bad hour. And she said that he probably wouldn't survive.

Nicholas did survive, and Graciela's family interpreted this good fortune to be the result of their immediate action. Fredrico acted upon common knowledge that eggs can be used to draw out negative energy, and subsequently turned to a curandera for further help (for more on the curative power of eggs, see Hunt, 1992, p. 49; Rubel, 1960, pp. 800–801). As this example shows, traditional medicine continues to provide meaningful explanations of and responses to illness in contemporary life, and Graciela's words highlight the way in which caregivers might turn to traditional healers to attend to elders' immediate needs.

As discussed in the previous chapter, "traditional" (or natural) medicine does not refer to a codified system but rather a general orientation of physical and spiritual health that emphasizes equilibrium among individual, social, and ecological domains (Rubel, 1960). In contrast to Western tendencies that separate mind from body, traditional medicine does not have a mind-body division and sees health as an expression of the harmonious functioning of the whole organism (Rubel & Browner, 1999). Moreover, when anthropologists and clinicians refer to traditional medicine, they also reference the shared and constructed knowledge of the local environment's curative properties (for example, medicinal plants, healthy foods, therapeutic benefits of being in nature, and so forth), and the larger social role held by healers in their respective communities (Sesia, 1996).

As Valentina Napolitano (2002) writes of her own study on medical pluralism in Mexico, "Complementary [that is, traditional] medicines are part of a postmodern condition" that are not a vestige of the past, but "an emergent phenomenon that re-inscribes tradition into modernity" (p. 105). Indeed, this fact is even inherent in the historical roots of traditional medicine. In the previous chapter, I wrote that however much traditional medicine might imply something in reference to "traditional" culture, it does not actually originate from "pure" pre-Hispanic origins, but is rather representative of Mexico's broader syncretic history that combined humoral theory (introduced by the Spaniards) as well as other abroad sources.[4] This variegated system became formalized into a distinct medical practice during the colonial period, distinguished in comparison to the humoral medical system legitimized by the Spaniards. The most recognized traditional practitioner is the curandera, an expert with specialized knowledge who works to diagnose sites of disequilibrium and reestablish harmony (Ortiz et al., 2008; Treviño, 2001; J. C. Young & Garro, 1993).[5] Yet however much curanderas are often described as general practitioners in other Mexican settings, in Teotitlán they are perceived with more specificity. The Zapotec word for curandera—benny ni rusiak dxiby—translates as "person who cures susto." This means that, at least nominally, curanderas are not perceived as medical practitioners in a general sense, but as having expertise in a very specified arena. Curanderas are individuals who possess specialized knowledge about local plants and herbs, and use this knowledge for the treatment of susto. They administer teas and provide other traditional interventions (incantations, limpias [spiritual cleansings], card divination, and more). Nevertheless, and despite the specificity that this name conveys in Teotitlán, their practice is supple and wide-ranging. Through my fieldwork I came across cases of curanderas being consulted for *mal de ojo* (evil eye), hora mala, *pérdida del alma* (soul loss), spirit possession, divination, the common cold, and other maladies.[6]

Throughout Oaxaca and Mexico, curanderas and traditional medicine in general have been indexed against broader notions of social progress. Individuals experience stigma talking about their use of traditional medicine, and it has been documented in Mexico City that more than 64 percent of patients did not report their use of traditional remedies to their physician (Argaez-Lopez et al., 2003). This sensibility extends to individuals in Oaxaca and is expressive of Mexico's broader history that incorporated and delimitated traditional medical practices. Well after the Spanish attempted to eradicate indigenous medicine, during Mexico's 1910 revolution, indigenous cultures were seen as an obstacle to efforts to the new nationalism that sought to *"mestizo-ize"* (whiten) the indigenous population. *Indigenismo* was a core feature of revolutionary and postrevolutionary ideology, centering on an idea of Mexican national identity that romanticized indigenous culture as Mexico's origin, while, in so doing, created a construct of the "Indian" as a figure of the past and at odds with modernity (Knight, 1990; Lewis, 2006). This widely impacted the prevalence and perception of traditional medicine. For example, until the 1970s, national policy written by the Instituto Nacional Indigenista (National Indigenous Institute) aimed to eradicate indigenous healers and discourage traditional medical treatment (see Duncan, 2017b, p. 44). This reversed in conjunction with other national and international policies that began to promote multiculturalism. Culminating in the 1994 Zapatista movement that put indigenous issues in the political spotlight, national policy shifted to recognize Mexico as a multicultural nation with varied social (including medical) practices. For example, in comparison to the 1970s government policy, a recent report written by the National Health Secretary writes that the national government "respects the free decision of citizens in choosing which medical model meets their needs" (Secretaría de Salud, 2007, p. 23). And similarly, since 2001 with the passage of Oaxaca's Decreto 345, the state has come to recognize traditional medicine as a legitimate practice on the same legal footing as biomedicine (Gutmann, 2007, p. 190). Yet these public policies have not translated to tangible cultural change. As Whitney Duncan (2018), Mathew Gutmann (2007), and Paola Sesia (1996) have shown in their respective research in Oaxaca, viewing traditional medicine as a "right" is different than it standing on par with biomedicine, and traditional medicine continues to be viewed with stigma and is associated to cultural "backwardness" in implicit reference to indigenismo ideology.

This helps account for today's varied appeal of traditional medicine in Teotitlán. Households like Graciela's justified their decision to consult traditional specialists in reference to how traditional medicine is indexed to cultural identity. In Mario's words, "We took him to the curandera because that's our first choice before taking him to a doctor. . . . We took him to the curandera because it was susto." Mario's comments draw attention to how curanderas are called upon because they are perceived to treat a certain category of illness that physicians cannot. Curanderas treat spiritual attacks that are considered different than physical ailments. In this way, medical systems are distinguished not only because of their ability to provide varying medical interventions, but also because of their ability to detect varying illness categories (see also Ayora-Diaz, 1998, p. 166; Higgins, 1975, p. 35; Hunt, 1992; Napolitano, 2002; Whiteford, 1995; J. C. Young & Garro, 1993).

But for caregivers like Graciela and family, recognizing these symptoms as a case of susto is also an implicit stance that affirms traditional perspectives over more "modern" ones. This was apparent when Graciela and family told me that the treatment provided by the curandera actually took a long time to take effect, and also when Mario's wife, Isabelle, discussed the treatment Nicholas received, and why it was meaningful to the family:

> What the curandera uses are materials from the earth like water, rocks, fire, and everything that belongs to the earth. And that's how they work—just like our ancestors used to work. And that's one of the reasons why we took him there, before taking him to a doctor. Because something else might happen to him that might be cured by a curandera. . . . [And so] she prescribed a natural medicine—she prepared some herbs for him to drink, and she left us some herbs to make drinks for him. And he was cleansed with an egg, and we were told to throw away the egg very far [because it contained dangerous energy].

Isabelle's description provides a glimpse of how curanderas work, but also about the way their work is perceived to serve as a bridge between idealized notions about cultural origin and modern experience. Curiously, after the family states that the curandera was slow to ameliorate Nicholas's symptoms, their description is nevertheless positive. They describe how curanderas use time-honored remedies, "just like our ancestors," and express that this is their first choice when seeking medical assistance. This is not just a description of traditional medicine, but also a justification of it. The family turns to traditional medicine *because* it is part and parcel of their views of cultural identity.

During my research I had the opportunity to meet Juanita, a curandera who also happened to care for her husband recovering from a series of debilitating strokes. In her practice, Juanita worked from home and gained recognition in the community for treating cases of epilepsy. She was also proud of curing an individual from Mexico City temporarily residing in Teotitlán who did not initially believe in traditional medicine but was nevertheless cured from symptoms involving abrupt weight loss and fearfulness. Juanita understood this to be a case of susto related to his being victim of a highway robbery. She treated him with a series of local plants, and also advised him to return to the site of the robbery. Within weeks, he regained his health. Similar to Graciela's experience, after the stroke Juanita witnessed in her own husband, she noticed that he could hardly speak or ambulate. Juanita drew upon local understandings of illness regarding disequilibrium and also explained that her husband's condition resulted from psychological stress. "I believe it was due to a lot of stress and the anger that he had. That's what I believe caused everything. And I think it goes back to his childhood." Juanita explained how a dispute between her husband and his father about who would inherit the family property rendered the family disjointed and her husband experiencing stress throughout his life. Throughout their marriage, she tried to convince her husband to go on walks and engage with their own children, implicitly reinvoking the sense of family that he felt he had lost with his parents. And, though after his first stroke, Juanita and her husband consulted physicians at the Centro de Salud and later a neurologist, they found the medications they received to be ineffective. "The doctor's medication didn't work. And even now, I don't think it's working. So I plan to start giving him natural medicines so he can get better. That's why I take walks with him." Although she knows her husband is not suffering from susto, Juanita said that related medicines will likely be effective toward treating his condition. She described local plants—respective ones for men and women—and how she uses them in conjunction with other remedies, like walking in nature, limpias, and other restorative measures. At once, Juanita's approach illustrates how traditional medicine is viewed as an alternative to biomedical options, as well as how it leads to locally meaningful responses to social disequilibrium.

Similar to how susto and traditional medical concepts are a matter of belief for Graciela and Juanita, *not* pursuing traditional medicine is analogously related to disbelief. Over and over, among different caregivers and across various households (and also with other individuals I surveyed in the community), I encountered the same statement: people (do not) visit curanderas as a matter of belief. Whenever traditional medicine was discussed, people invoked the Zapotec word *relilaz*, "to believe" (for example, *"Kety relilaza rumedy kan,"* meaning "I don't believe in that treatment"). Yet as anthropologists have noted, justifying (or dismissing) something as a matter of belief carries subtle implications. Pouillon (2016) reminds us that the notion of belief is "paradoxical in that it expresses doubt as well as assurance" (p. 485). To say that one believes in something implies a conviction, but it also conveys awareness of doubt about that conviction. To further this point, Byron Good (1996) turns to etymology to highlight how belief is a "modern idea" that differs from its original meaning. Originally, writes Good, the concept of belief was linked to notions of affection and a relationship with something held dear, and only later came to imply a presupposition tentatively held to be true in contrast to higher, absolute knowledge (pp. 15–17). That is why today, across many cultures, to say one "believes" in a given entity like medicine means something different than saying one has "knowledge" of it; the former is marked by tentative faith and the latter by unwavering certitude.[7]

In medically plural settings like Teotitlán, this semantic dichotomy is adapted to rationalize the difference between "traditional" and "modern" medicines, where the notion of belief is used to describe traditional medicine, and knowledge is used in reference to biomedicine. This distinction creates a further division among how epistemological claims imply and divide various geographical territories. Curanderas are seen to work in a setting concerned with local dimensions of human life—drawing on local medicinal knowledge, local illness concepts, and local ecological harmony—while allopathic doctors, in comparison, are trained in institutions that represent the modern world and have access to universal knowledge purported to transcend the local. When *belief* is appealed to justify traditional medicine, it is done so in the context of (and in contrast to) the wide-ranging authority biomedicine has over local perspectives. And, conversely, as Stacy Pigg (1996) acutely observes in her own fieldwork in a different setting, claiming to *not believe* in traditional medicine only makes sense if you have somewhere else to go—namely, the modern, cosmopolitan world.

This epistemological dichotomy is present throughout Teotitlán, both among caregivers who profess to believe in traditional medicine and those who deny it. For example, in his experience caring for his wife with a finger amputation and Alzheimer's disease, Carlos and his adult son, Francisco, highlighted an interesting intergenerational disagreement about their respective beliefs about traditional medicine.

> CARLOS: I'm not very into natural medicines. And [I know how] we live nowadays [is different, but] natural medicine worked before. But also it killed a lot of people. And also a lot of people lived because of it. And when it works, it works slowly. Compared to the doctor's [medicine], it's quicker. That's why I'm not really into natural medicine.
>
> FRANCISCO: No, we're not into it. [*Moments later Francisco adds:*] We don't really believe in that.

For Carlos it is not the case that traditional medicine is ineffective. He clearly states that he knows it can work (albeit slowly). Yet he also recognizes that it can cause harm. But these comments are not merely about medical efficacy per se; they rather point toward a broader idea about the community to explain why traditional medicine is not utilized. Life has changed. The circumstances of living in Teotitlán are different such that traditional medicine and traditional illness categories no longer seem relevant. This is what Carlos means when he says that it "worked before" and when he compares it to "the way we live nowadays." Carlos's comments stand in contrast to his son, Francisco, a generation younger, who affirms that traditional medicine is not something he or his family believe in at all. Indeed, whereas Carlos implies he *does* believe in traditional medicine, Francisco's concluding words highlight generational difference about how traditional medicine is perceived as something relegated to the cultural past. To further understand this point, I inquired whether concepts like soul loss could be mobilized to explain the severe forgetfulness Francisco observed in his mother. "No, that's not the case," Francisco said. "Because if it were the case we would have visited a natural healer. But this is just not the case." This further builds on Francisco's comments regarding how traditional illness categories are no longer relevant. If he happened to believe that his mother's forgetfulness owed to soul loss (or a related traditional illness category), then he would have sought relevant help. But he does not. Hence, Francisco explains, curanderas are relevant for treating traditional illnesses, but it is only that those illnesses are believed to no longer exist.

Francisco's professed disbelief in traditional medicine is further revealing of local dynamics given the prevalence of nonbiomedical ideas about illness (for example, the way that he was shown in the previous chapter to understand the stress related to his mother's amputation as being the cause of her severe forgetfulness). Indeed, ideas alternative to biomedicine permeate most understandings of forgetfulness. Yet many caregivers also stopped short of endorsing traditional illness categories like susto or pérdida del alma. Perhaps one reason for this is accounted for through the logic of belief. Like Francisco stated, *if* he believed, he would go. There is a commitment implied in this statement, and for this reason he does not believe. Similar to Stacy Pigg (1996), who writes in her study of shamans in Nepal, "your attitude towards shamans communicates who you are" (p. 160), one's attitude toward curanderas in Oaxaca involves the negotiation of what modernity means, and how individuals decide to position themselves in regard to it and concomitant notions of tradition. This sheds further light on the way traditional medicine is indexed to broader stigma that some Teotitecos attempt to navigate and avoid. Francisco's statement that he does not believe in traditional medicine is situated in this understanding.

Indeed, there were many instances during my fieldwork when I was told by acquaintances that they did not believe in traditional medicine, only to later find out they had recently consulted a curandera for specific illnesses. People seemed to experience stigma and embarrassment for engaging with traditional medicine—and perhaps even more upon talking about this subject with me, a foreigner to the community. Yet this shows how individuals' avoidance of traditional medicine is embedded within broader power structures that render health-seeking choices into a matter of belief, maintained in juxtaposition to biomedicine. In the process, traditional medicine becomes a symbol of backwardness or the maintenance of local identity—depending on one's belief—highlighting the perceived tension between ideals concerning local tradition and modern life.

BIOMEDICAL OPTIONS: "THAT'S WHEN THEY TOLD ME THAT THERE IS THIS DISEASE"

The night of Nicholas's first stroke, his family thought he was dead. After appearing disheveled and unable to speak, Nicholas grew immobile and eventually lost vital signs of life. "He looked like he was dying," Mario said. And Isabelle added, while standing over the loom and taking a break from the rug she had been weaving:

> He *was* dead—when we touched him, he wasn't breathing at all, his blood wasn't circulating, his nose wasn't passing air. He got

cold, and that's when we realized what it was. So [my husband and brother-in-law] took him to the Centro de Salud [Teotitlán's local hospital], but our assumption was that he got scared of something. That's what we believe in.

This was their first description of what happened that fateful night, and it took time to piece together the details of how Graciela's family came to bring Nicholas to the local hospital. Because they believed Nicholas was suffering from susto, they initially sought help from a curandera. But they were later advised by this healer to go to the hospital. "We took him to the curandera because that's our first choice before taking him to a doctor," Mario said. "However, afterward we went to the doctor because she told us to take him." Indeed, while allopathic providers might be averse in referring patients to "alternative" treatments because of stigma, I came across other similar instances where curanderas advised families to visit doctors.[8] In this case, Nicholas was first treated by the curandera for susto, and was subsequently referred to visit the hospital for high blood pressure. As Graciela's family made clear, both providers were seen as integral to keeping Nicholas alive.

In Teotitlán allopathic doctors are locally known and respected individuals who have specialized knowledge to cure illness. The Zapotec term for doctor, *benny ni rusiak*, literally means "a person who cures." As this phrase suggests, doctors are known to treat a variety of ailments and have been present in Teotitlán for centuries, embedded in extended histories of conquest, colonialism and, as I will continue to argue, contemporary regimes of power.

The arrival of the Spaniards who conquered Oaxaca in 1521 signified what Kristen Norget (2006) rightly calls "cultural rupture," shattering and displacing dominated orders of meaning, and remaking the entire sociopolitical landscape (p. 91). While the actual conquest of Oaxaca lasted just under one week—and the Zapotecs capitulated without engaging in battle—the consequences were devastating (Murphy & Stepick, 1991, p. 16; see also Mathew, Mathew, & Oudijk, 2007). The Conquistadores introduced what has perhaps been the region's most devastating weapon—measles, smallpox, typhus, and other infectious diseases against which the indigenous population had no immunity. The numbers alone are staggering, giving pause for the magnitude of losses. Whereas at the eve of the Conquest there were an estimated 350,000 indigenous people living in Oaxaca Valley, by 1568 the population dwindled to 150,000 and, by 1630 only 40,000 remained—a 90 percent drop in less than a 100-year period (Murphy & Stepick, 1991, p. 18).

This history also significantly impacted local medical practice. While Span-iards were initially fascinated by the knowledge indigenous populations had accumulated of medicinal plants, they soon came to prohibit much of it because they found it threatening and heretical.[9] From the time of the Conquest, the Spaniards introduced European-trained *médicos*, whose practice was initially based on classical Greek humoral medical theory. As already discussed, these practi-tioners and other Conquistadores challenged and eventually subverted indige-nous medical treatment, leading to the eventual undermining of pre-Hispanic medicine as a legitimate treatment option (Somolinos d'Ardois, 1976; Treviño, 2001, p. 54). Nevertheless, New World physicians began to selectively incor-porate humoral medicine with parts of what remained of local knowledge of medicinal plants, leading to a *mestizo* (mixed) medical practice (Hernández Sáenz & Foster, 2001, pp. 19–25). This persisted until the early nineteenth century, when French-based biomedicine was introduced to Mexico, leading to the contemporary dominant approach that emphasizes objectivity through distin-guishing between underlying observable (biological) causes and subjective (psychosocial) experiences of illness.

Today, the purported objectivity associated with biomedical knowledge stands in contrast to the beliefs people have toward traditional medicine. Biomed-icine has come to be defined by a specific orientation that posits illness to have underlying, universal features, and medical knowledge as objectively accounting for those features. Yet however much we take biomedicine to be an objective "mirror of nature," it is a cultural activity like any other social phenomenon, constituted by specific outlooks and values. Yes, biomedicine is able to make critical observations that I do not wish to dismiss. But these observations are also steeped within cultural values that shape how people interpret and respond to them. As Good (1996) argues, we have been seduced into thinking that biomedical "knowledge" is somehow less cultural and contingent than traditional "belief," and thus fail to appreciate how biomedicine is also socially constructed; in the United States, he argues, biomedicine is often situated within notions of salvation and purity and linked to broader forms of state power. This is Foucault's (1975) point when he reminds us that the purported objectivity of the "clinical gaze" did not arise from technological innovation or the unavoidable development of a neutral standpoint—from simply detecting somatic signs that were waiting to be seen. Rather, Foucault argues, the clinical gaze originated from within a specific cultural epoch that prioritized depth such that it made sense to detect underlying signs of illness. Again, the point is not to dismiss the unquestionable utility and efficacy of biomedicine, but to situate it within a specific cultural landscape and unsettle the way it is commonly viewed to be objective and free from cultural influence.

In Mexico, congruent with how traditional medicine is linked to notions of backwardness, biomedicine is indexed to notions of economic development and social modernization. State campaigns meant to raise public awareness about health care invariably aim to also instill citizens with "modern" health behaviors that facilitate economic and social ends (Wentzell, 2015). This is written in federal policy as, for example, when the National Health Secretary has extended concern about health to include mental health whose "importance . . . [is recognized] not only as a health issue, but also because of its impact on socioeconomic development for nations" (Secretaría de Salud, 2001, p. 13; see also Duncan, 2017b). Linking health to development testifies to how biomedicine is contextualized within national efforts toward "modernization" and, conversely, how choosing to forgo biomedical intervention is viewed as a larger stance against national progress.

As I began to collect and compare stories like Graciela's family decision to send Nicholas to the Centro de Salud to treat high blood pressure, I came to recognize that no household consulted a physician for forgetfulness itself, but rather because of other somatic complaints. This highlighted telling perspectives of biomedicine's social power, as well as how it comes to introduce new perspectives of age-related forgetfulness. Alberto, Beatrice, and Cecilia (the caregivers discussed in chapter 2 whose mother was diagnosed with osteoporosis and senile dementia) reflected on how they came to learn their mother had an illness pertaining to forgetfulness when they had initially considered forgetfulness normal. Beatrice explained why they initially turned to a doctor:

> It was because of the pain in her feet, and her knees, her waist, and she would always complain about her pain. Everything happened gradually. It first started with her feet, then she used a cane. And then the cane wasn't able to support her weight anymore, so she used a walker. And then we thought that the pain was probably in her knee. And then we took her to the doctor and he told us that she had severe osteoporosis. And he said that she needed a study, but the study she needed was for her whole body [including her brain]. So then they realized that she had [senile dementia]. And they asked her some questions. According to the answer of the questions, they also diagnosed the illness she has [that is, senile dementia].

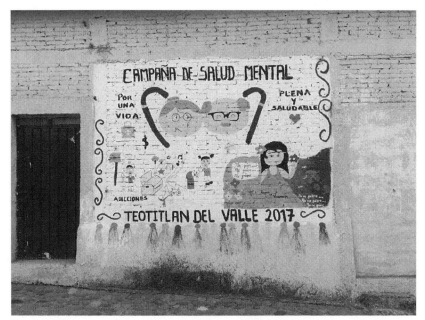

FIG. 3.1. Though this mural was found after the majority of fieldwork occurred, it provides further illustration of how mental health is situated as a matter of public health. The mural coalesces many themes about modern lifestyles—self-love that moderates risk of domestic abuse, that exercising, recycling, remaining mentally active, and being compliant with medical check-ups are important—and how these activities all lead to healthy aging. Further illustrating how these paths are situated within broader notions of modernity, the mural coalesces around a depiction of two Caucasian elders who have attained the goal. *Photograph by the author.*

In light of the fact that this household viewed forgetfulness as nonproblematic, Alberto and his family did not visit a doctor because of it. Instead, they initially sought consultation because of the elder's pain. At first tolerable, the elder's pain increasingly grew more acute such that at a decisive point, they decided to seek medical help. It was the moment they suspected that the elder's pain was located in her knee—pain with a hypothesized physical origin—that they made the decision to seek help. This line of reasoning illustrates a preliminary reason for why doctors are considered useful—they cure pain that has a physical origin, resonating with prior research that shows how other Mexican indigenous communities perceive doctors as treating physical, not mental or spiritual, ailments (Ayora-Diaz, 1998). But, in the process of visiting the doctor to treat

Juana's knee, the consultation ends with an answer to a question they had not
raised. It was through visiting a doctor for somatic pain that the family learns
about senile dementia, an illness wholly different from her presenting problem.

Whereas Alberto and his family consulted a doctor because of physical pain,
caregivers also consulted doctors because of knowledge about other somatic
symptoms that did not involve pain at all. Pablo and Vanessa were caregivers
briefly discussed in previous chapters, a married couple who care for an elder
diagnosed with Alzheimer's disease. They similarly described how they consulted
a physician for symptoms not related to forgetfulness and came to learn the
elder had Alzheimer's disease. Vanessa described why they initially turned to
a physician:

> Because of her high blood pressure, that's why we took her. . . . That's
> when they asked her [if she was taking her medication]. And at that
> time I already knew that she wasn't taking the medication anymore. . . .
> And so when I took her to the clinic, she told the doctor that she was
> still taking her medicine. That's when they [the doctors] realized that
> she forgets. And that's when they told me that there is this disease that's
> called [Alzheimer's disease], and perhaps that's what she has.

This excerpt again demonstrates that forgetfulness is not caregivers' reason to
seek medical help. Vanessa's description mirrors much of what Beatrice says—
even how the diagnosis pertaining to forgetfulness is discovered accidentally.
But here Vanessa reveals that there exist other symptoms that lead caregivers
to seek help. Previous awareness about high blood pressure—and Vanessa's
knowledge that medical doctors are the appropriate individuals to treat this
condition—justified their visit.

The observation that caregivers visit doctors for reasons other than forgetfulness holds, even for more severe cases. Caring for his wife with Alzheimer's
who had "completely" forgotten, Carlos and his son Francisco described how
their attentiveness to his wife's thinking too much after her finger amputation
led them to consult a physician. Francisco explained:

> Well, she started to forget very often. And consequently her behavior
> wasn't normal anymore. . . . What depressed her the most was that she
> lost a finger. [And] due to that situation, it started to get worse. . . . So
> we took her to a neurologist [because of the depression]. . . . Yes, he is
> the one that diagnosed her with Alzheimer's.

Here, Carlos and his family are aware of forgetfulness—they know that the elder has begun to forget in a concerning, not "normal" way—but their decision to visit a doctor is again not due to forgetfulness in itself. They visited a neurologist for the elder's sadness and, again, it is through this encounter they learned that she has Alzheimer's disease.[10] The family's turn to a physician for mental health concerns (and Pablo and Vanessa's turn for high blood pressure) illustrate how medical doctors are perceived to treat nonphysical symptoms beyond somatic pain—and also how these consultations lead to new perspectives of forgetfulness itself.

In each of these instances it is instructive to note that no caregiver thought to consult a doctor because of memory complaints—nor did they consider visiting a doctor to assess memory—but elders nevertheless left being diagnosed with an illness concerning it. In a setting where doctors are not the only individuals known to cure illness, one must pause and consider the vast power this shows them to have. Indeed, whereas indigenous (or traditional) medicines have been historically delegitimized through ruling dominations, biomedical practice continues to be embedded and reaffirmed through government programs, standardized medical procedures, and broader economic and political parameters. Teotitlán's Centro de Salud is symbolically situated at this powerful center, at the base of the community's main arterial motorway to serve the Teotiteco and neighboring communities. Many of the doctors are not from Teotitlán, but other parts of Mexico, and are carrying out temporary residency programs. These doctors are consulted through routine to monitor somatic complaints—conditions like high blood pressure and diabetes.[11] Yet for the majority in Teotitlán who receive a pension, this is not a personal choice one makes, but something required by government policy. The government-sponsored pension program, 70 y Más, gives elders a pension *on the condition that* they biannually visit doctors and attend bimonthly *pláticas* (informational workshops on biomedical health and treatment; see also Sesia, 2001).[12] (A similar pension program, Prospera [formerly Oportuni-dades] provides financial support for the rest of the population meeting poverty criteria in exchange for regular health-care visits and information sessions.) In so doing, the state legitimizes and transforms one medical system over another, illustrating how power relations shape healing in local contexts (see also Connor, 2001, p. 4; Menéndez, 1994; Rose, 2007). The power represented by allopathic providers at once demonstrates the regularity and legitimization of medical consultation—what Foucault (1984) calls the "politics of health"—and the way biomedical information about conditions like diabetes and Alzheimer's disease is circulated as a matter of public concern. Moreover, it illustrates limitations in explaining health-seeking behavior as solely motivated by a pragmatism for what is best for elders. Yes, the decision to seek medical help is, in part, motivated by caregivers' pragmatic concern to ensure elders' well-being and to attend to the broader cohesion of the family unit. Yet these encounters also reveal how health-seeking behavior is simultaneously constituted within broader power structures that influence with whom and how consultations occur.

These observations go beyond initial visits with physicians and include their recommendations for follow-up care. After Graciela and her sons took Nicholas to the Centro de Salud to address his high blood pressure, they were advised to go to a specialist in Oaxaca City for further diagnostic testing. Mario said, "They told us that we had to have a study on him in Oaxaca. But they also told us that all they would be able to tell us is what's wrong with his brain and that he wasn't going to get any better. And that [the study] is going to be expensive." Like other households, when caregivers consult local doctors, they are given a tentative diagnosis that they are then told can only be confirmed through subsequent consultation with a specialist. This was a consistent finding across all the households I interviewed who had met with a doctor who had suspected or diagnosed dementia. In Graciela's case, she and her family decided to forgo the tests, reasoning that the additional knowledge that they would have gained about Nicholas's condition did not justify the financial burden they would incur in the process.

While previous research has shown that health-seeking behavior among populations with dementia is related to cultural outlooks on forgetfulness (Hinton, Franz, & Friend, 2004), this perspective alone is insufficient to address the structural determinants that contextualize what these decisions entail. Like how Graciela and her family reasoned that it was not financially viable to see a specialist in Oaxaca City, many other households held similar rationales that weighed on whether receiving a definitive diagnosis from a specialist would improve how they provided care. For example, Pablo and Vanessa had a similar experience upon their visit to the Centro de Salud. In Pablo's words, "They told us that if we took her to a specialist, we could be certain. But . . . we're doing the best we can. And to take her to a specialist is more expensive." And later he clarified what sort of information he could be certain of, as he hoped to afford a visit with a specialist in the future:

> Well first of all, we'll get our questions answered, and what probability
> [she has to recover]. . . . I hope that he will tell us the truth, whether

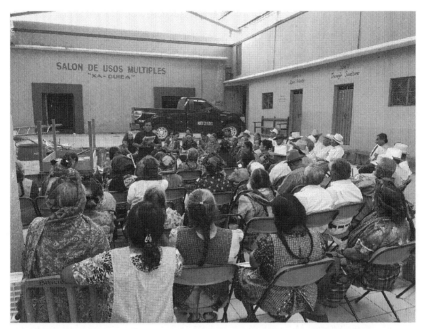

Fig. 3.2. *Plática* (informational health workshop). Domingo Gutierrez Mendoza, the local organizer of Teotitlán's 70 y Más, leads a workshop for elders about nutrition. *Photograph by the author.*

it's really because of her age that she cannot get better, and if it's going to get worse until the day she passes away. Or if there is a way to save her if I had the money. Those are the questions I want answered. But I'm hoping to have money in the near future. . . . Even if I don't buy the medication [the doctor might prescribe], at least I'd get my questions answered.

Pablo's words shed light onto the way specialized doctors are perceived and the type of services they are thought to provide. Though Pablo and his family cannot afford it, they speculate on how specialists might offer more-definitive diagnostic answers than general doctors. He begins to wonder about the expected course of Alzheimer's, and whether there might be available medications or other treatment options. He wants this information so he can know how to plan for the future and also so that he might provide better care. But he knows it is out of his financial means. This brings up the resources Pablo knows are available—but just not to people like him with financial limitations, further highlighting structural economic inequalities implicit within everyday caregiving experience. In the end, although Pablo suspects that specialists could help, and although he personally wants to consult one, he and his family decide to not pursue this option. These comments also point toward how biomedicine is locally understood to hold a perspective of truth that might stand at odds with other, traditional perspectives. "I hope that he will tell us the truth," implies that specialists and, by extension, allopathic doctors have access to an underlying truth about illness that might not otherwise be known. Believing that the truth about illness exists—despite not being able to financially access it—is a stance that highlights one medical system at the expense of the other. It again reveals the local difference between "belief" and "knowledge," where physicians hold epistemological authority over other medical traditions. But here, even when that authority is recognized, biomedicine is perceived within financial constraints that limit Pablo's ability to pursue it.

In addition to financial reasons, caregivers also chose not to consult (specialist or generalist) physicians because it was against what elders wanted for themselves. This came up during a conversation with Sergio, Manuel, and Linda about why they have yet to gain diagnostic clarification about Pedro's progressively impactful forgetfulness.

> Linda: No, he hasn't been diagnosed with anything because he doesn't want to go.
>
> Sergio: He doesn't want to go to the doctor. And even if he were to go, if they were to prescribe any medications, he would just take it all at once. So I don't see how there's a point to take him to the doctor since he won't take his medications the way he's supposed to.

Despite the fact that Sergio's father cannot recall his name, and the risks involved in Pedro's dangerous tendency to wander, Sergio and his family decide not to consult a doctor—or any medical specialist. Their reason is simple: Pedro does not want it. This helps show how, even if caregivers were interested in consulting doctors, they overlook their own desires in order to honor what elders want.[13] Though this decision may appear to be a negation of caregiving responsibilities, there is also good reason to understand it as a mechanism that upholds them. In light of how I have discussed Teotiteco family structure, research on Latino elders shows that social and familial support is more important to elders' sense of well-being than medical attention (Beyene, Becker, & Mayen, 2002). Hence, by respecting elders' wishes not to visit a doctor, caregivers are perceived as attending to them in a significant way.[14] Sergio and his family highlight how listening to elders and demonstrating respect—and, in some instances, eclipsing their own inclinations to seek professional help—is central caregiving itself.

To further illustrate this perspective, I return to my research on Alberto, Beatrice, and Cecilia. Although these caregivers had consulted a general doctor for osteoporosis and subsequently learned Juana had senile dementia, their decision to not consult a medical specialist further illustrates how doctors might be considered irrelevant because the problems elders face are seen as a standard feature of aging. Similar to other caregivers who speculated on the help a medical specialist might provide, at one point Alberto said, "If we took her to a specialist, they might help. But she says that that's the way she's decided to end her life. When we tell her to visit the doctor she answers, 'There's no need for me to go to the doctor—I'm old.' " Alberto speculates that a medical specialist might be able to help, but nevertheless he and his family choose to not consult one. This again casts further light on the pragmatism I observed in the previous chapter. Whereas earlier I argued that caregivers assume a stance that opens up possibilities for action to provide for elders, here Alberto demonstrates an instance where he and his family deliberately decide to not take action. As Alberto explains, this decision is made in light of his mother's resounding statement, "I'm old." This is a conviction that forgetfulness is a natural feature of aging, and a signifier for how aging invokes progressive loss. Doctors are here for treating illness when it is not supposed to happen, but aging is a process where illness is expected. Hence, another reason not to visit a doctor concerns representations of aging and the way in which illness is understood to inescapably accompany this part of the lifecycle. There is more involved in one's decision to seek medical care than just simple pragmatism to do what is best.

The most obvious impact medical consultations have is the way in which they transform "normal" forgetfulness into a diagnosed biomedical disease. This is representative of what Carroll Estes and Elizabeth Binney (1989) term the "biomedicalization of aging," a process whereby perceived normal physical and mental decline is placed under the domain and control of biomedicine.[15] All of the caregivers who consulted doctors made their decisions on the basis of previously known biomedical illness categories, or because visits were required by the state's pension program. Yet in the process, they were introduced to a new illness category—senile dementia, Alzheimer's disease, stroke, or vascular dementia—thereby expanding the scope and power of biomedicine. This finding, implicit throughout the previous pages, is important with regard to how the perception of elders is changing in Teotitlán. Following Duncan (2018), who observes how Oaxacan mental health professionals go beyond the provision of treatment to actively foment local culture change in the way mental health is understood and pursued, the above discussion demonstrates how doctors, nurses, and other stakeholders in biomedicine are equally integral to a type of "cultural change"—now, initiating not only a change in the scope of biomedical practice, but a more fundamental reconstruction of how the aging process is understood.

~

This chapter has advanced a number of observations about the choices caregivers face in engaging with medical specialists. The implicit distinction between "knowledge" in biomedicine and "belief" in traditional medicine presupposes power structures that legitimize one system at the expense of the other. Health-seeking decisions are rooted in epistemological assumptions and reveal how the way things are held to be true is structured by broader social, political, and economic factors. This is not only based in perceptual differences made between medical systems, but broader idealized notions of modernization and social progress. When caregivers choose to consult traditional medical providers, they do so as part of a larger stance that engages with notions of tradition and local identity in the context of modern alternatives. Conversely, when caregivers consult biomedical providers, this choice is representative of a larger affirmation of ideas about modernization. This latter perspective is rooted in the power attributed to biomedical providers—from historical perspectives that establish legitimacy to government policy and fiscal programs that require engagement. The regularity of consulting physicians comes to change how age-related forgetfulness is understood and contrasts with broader representations of aging that view illness as a normal part of the lifecycle.

As a whole, the choices that caregivers make in consulting physicians, specialists, and traditional healers concern—and are responsive to—factors that go beyond the provision of care, and involve broader ideas about how to maintain tradition in a setting perceived to be increasingly "modern." The medical pluralism described in this chapter is not just about a set of choices one has between different types of providers, but a broader "arena for the negotiation of social difference" (Pigg, 1995, p. 19). This is a negotiation situated between socioeconomic spectrums and cultural differences, and also between the opposite idealized poles represented by "tradition" and "modernity" that inscribe those differences, including the inhabited gray zones that most caregivers are situated in as they make medical choices. This marks the concrete difference that health-seeking behaviors entail, bringing us back to the pragmatists who remind us that what we take to be true (or a sound medical decision) is not based on an objective reading of the world, but rather a perspective that is furnished based on its usefulness. Things become useful in specific cultural worlds as they are inscribed by broader realms of power that influence what is taken to be valuable and true. In this way, the dichotomy between beliefs about traditional medicine and knowledge of biomedicine are cultural expressions, rendered meaningful and distinct in a world where one is legitimized at the expense of the other. Just as truth is made rather than found, caregivers' medical decisions engage with broader concerns about how they negotiate elements of their cultural heritage in a world perceived to be increasingly modern.

The negotiation of social difference inherent in health-seeking decisions is also part of what constitutes the segregative component in my analysis of the segre-social dynamics of caregiving. As social differences are negotiated between medical systems, so too are decisions about how to engage with (or jettison) idealized notions of communal heritage, and the subsequent way caregivers are held accountable for their decisions. It could be argued that caregivers' health-seeking decisions help put into focus awareness of local identity and, by extension, provide a meaningful social space for how local identity is negotiated and redefined in the context of the tensions inherent to contemporary life. Traditional medicine is indexed not only to a cultural past that remains a historical constant, but to the meaning and function of the past as it dynamically adapts to the conditions of the present. In Teotitlán, each medical sector exists and is practiced in context of the other. Deciding to (not) consult providers from either sector is thus a moment of regenerating what it means to belong in the Teotiteco community and how to maintain values and traditions celebrated within it.

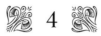

Relationships With Elders

CAREGIVING CHALLENGES, STRATEGIES,
AND PERCEPTIONS OF FORGETFUL ELDERS

"Elders are a very important part of society," Vanessa said while reflecting on her experience caregiving. "Why? Because they are old, they have life experience. But at the same time, they can behave just like children." During their two years of caregiving for Maria, an 85-year-old widow diagnosed with Alzheimer's disease, Vanessa and her husband, Pablo, have developed a perspective of aging that stands in contrast to how elders tend to be revered in the broader community. Their experience testifies to a tension between the ideal of the elder as *bengul*—a figure respected for accumulated life experience and wisdom—and the reality of how forgetful elders come to be viewed through the caregiving process. This tension is the theme of the present chapter as I seek to explore the everyday challenges, strategies, and relationships with elders that constitute caregiving experience.

So much of this tension was made evident through the ambivalence Pablo and Vanessa expressed about the way they became caregivers. When we first met, Pablo announced himself through the wrought-iron front gate of his home. His face was half shaded beneath a worn and splintering sombrero, and he was on his way to farm in the mountains. He and Vanessa were in their midforties, and had three young children who, out of curiosity, peeked their heads to observe as we spoke about my research in their courtyard. Pablo and Vanessa had their own home, apart from Pablo's parents, but were located on adjacent property to the rest of Pablo's family. Pablo and Vanessa were middle-class weavers, with one loom for Vanessa to use at home while Pablo left to work for a local merchant outside. As they continued to remind me, caregiving was an additional responsibility on top of many others—and they expressed ambivalence about why they had accepted responsibility for Maria when they had so much else to worry about.

Much of this sentiment was centered on how they came to be caregivers for Maria because, they explained, she was not directly related to either of them. Pablo and Vanessa said they were doing an *obra de caridad* (act of charity, using this Spanish term while speaking in Zapotec) after immediate family members did not volunteer to assume responsibility. Indeed, while I was repeatedly told that in Teotitlán, elders do not have to worry about social support and who will take care of them should they become dependent, Pablo and Vanessa's household highlighted tangible limits to that normative claim.

Maria is the widow of Vanessa's deceased uncle (Vanessa's "aunt-in-law") and, as Vanessa explained, this rendered her on the fringes of the family tree. Maria was raised and married in Teotitlán, but she and her husband later moved to Mexico City early in their twenties. They migrated for the promise of a more secure economic future, but continued to experience poverty throughout their lives. They had no children and Maria sold candies on the street, while her husband, who had a long history of alcoholism, moved boxes at wholesale markets. "They were very poor," Vanessa summarized, and explained how, because of their poverty, Maria and her husband eventually decided to return to Teotitlán in their old age. Family promised them a plot of land and social support. But upon returning seven years ago, the family of Maria's husband withdrew their offer. Maria and her husband suddenly found that they had no land or home to start their new life, and so her husband returned to Mexico City to earn money. He passed away two months later. After his death, Maria's in-laws said it was not their responsibility to open their home to her because they were no longer relatives, and that she needed to live elsewhere. "She cried for a long time, every day, because of that," Vanessa said. "Because she was left with nothing . . . and because they kicked her out of their house."

Initially, the two families closest to Maria strategized about how to support her. Maria has a sister in town with her own family, and so Pablo and Vanessa made an agreement with them to hold joint responsibilities. Maria would be free to choose when she wanted to stay with her sister, or to live with Pablo and Vanessa. Pablo explained, "We initially agreed to take care of her, and the other part of her family agreed to take care of her as well. And whenever she wanted to go there or here, we would always be available. But now since she's started to have these problems, we're the ones that take care of her most of the time."

Indeed, in the past two years, Maria began to show increasing signs of forgetfulness that later became diagnosed as Alzheimer's disease. Pablo and Vanessa understood this to be the result of Maria thinking too much after becoming a widow and losing family support. But this only exacerbated Maria's problems. Her sister's family soon demonstrated that they were ill prepared and lacked motivation to take adequate care of her—insufficiently feeding her, provoking arguments, and not preventing her from wandering—so Pablo and Vanessa have now come to assume full responsibility.

Reallocating responsibility to their home has been far from easy, and caregiving has significantly impacted Pablo and Vanessa's lives. Similar to other caregiving households, Pablo and Vanessa wake up each morning to bathe Maria and prepare her breakfast. But Maria frequently forgets that she was fed and accuses Pablo and Vanessa of neglecting her. Maria says things that are off-topic, forgets where she is and how to recognize public landmarks, and also has a tendency to leave home and wander. She forgets where she places objects like clothing and the TV remote control, and accuses Pablo, Vanessa, and their children of stealing from her. "All of a sudden she just gets mad, and she starts to yell," Vanessa said while thinking about how she is so often accused of mistreatment. "All of this affects me."

Caregiving involves intimate changes to relationships. Standard across caregiving literature is the observation that fundamental changes occur in how family members relate to elders living with dementia (for example, Hargrave & Anderson, 2013; Mace & Rabins, 2011; Schulz, 2000). Pablo and Vanessa make sure that Maria eats, bathes, and does not get lost, given her tendency to wander. They curb their frustration when they are provoked, and they ameliorate Maria's anger when she is irritated. These everyday experiences significantly shift the nature of their relationship with Maria. But they also signify the way caregiving is inherently meaningful. Included even in the ambivalence Pablo and Vanessa expressed about how they came to assume responsibility for Maria was the recognition that they also found caregiving to give greater purpose to their lives. The challenges they faced taught them about human dependency, intergenerational relationships, and what it means to grow old in Teotitlán today.

That is why presenting caregiving as a practice that is merely difficult or burdensome is inadequate; it overlooks the way caregivers also identify and pursue basic values through this experience. Indeed, despite the challenges caregivers noted in their roles, across all households, I observed how caregiving was a responsibility that led to substantial, everyday meaning (see also Guarnaccia et al., 1992; Norris, Pratt, & Kuiack, 2003, p. 340; Tarlow, 2004).

Much of what constitutes caregiving experience is that it is simultaneously structured by and sustains values that matter and make life meaningful. There is truth in observations made by anthropologists like Arthur Kleinman (2009), who describe caregiving as a "defining moral practice . . . [of] solidarity with those in great need . . . a moral practice that makes caregivers, and at times even the care-receivers, more present and thereby fully human" (p. 293). Caregiving is a reminder of the contingency of human life: we all depend on—and provide for—others to survive.

Vanessa's comment that "elders can behave just like children" is expressive of this contingency, but it also is expressive of how her relationship with Maria has shifted. Her experience shows how caregiving practice has the potential to alter the meaning of old age and the way elders are valued in society. As Annemarie Mol (2008) reminds us, however much caregiving is guided by ideas about what good or virtuous human life looks like, in caregiving, such understandings of goodness and virtue are persistently "tinkered with" and adapted to find "more bearable ways of living in—or with—reality" (p. 46). Comparing elders to children—while acknowledging their accumulated wisdom—is an instance of such tinkering. It shows how the caregiving relationship is premised on affirming key values about human dependency that bring people together, and the way those values are encountered, questioned, and regenerated in the process.

This chapter explores the nature of this relationship and the way local values are regenerated in its context. It looks into the specific ways caregivers come to relate to elders, and how this is indicative of a shift in the way elders are perceived and valued in the household. While in this chapter I explore what the phenomenological tradition calls the "lived experience" of how caregiving represents a particular form of sociality with elders, I also implicitly draw upon more recent theoretical perspectives from psychological anthropology on human subjectivity to explore the ways "in which the collective and the individual are intertwined and run together and . . . intimately linked in an intersubjective matrix" (Biehl, Good, & Kleinman, 2007, p. 14).[1] Caregiving represents one such matrix, the site of a new sociality where interpersonal relations between

caregivers and elders are constituted within and contested against larger normative standards of aging. To appreciate the nature of this setting, we need to be
attentive not only to how this relationship is situated within domestic parameters
of the home, but also within broader economic and political circumstances,
normative expectations, and other forms of global influence outside the home.

In what follows I discuss how caregiving represents a novel relationship that
stands in contrast to how elders are normatively given respect and authority—
how, as Vanessa explained, forgetful elders are simultaneously viewed as socially
important persons with experience, and also dependents resembling children in
need of care. This tension provides additional perspective on the segre-social
dynamics inherent in caregiving, illustrating how providing care to a dependent
elder creates tension with larger normative expectations about how elders ought
to be viewed. To explore this, I divide the chapter into three sections. In the first,
I examine the daily challenges inherent to caregiving and assess how they are
perceived within and responsive to larger social dynamics. Next, I turn to review
how caregiving challenges lead to a new form of relating to elders, comparing
elders to children and initiating an instance of what gerontologists term "role
reversal" that must be understood in context to broader social outlooks. Last,
I explore specific strategies caregivers employ to care for forgetful elders, and
how these strategies embody a new form of intergenerational relations. As a
whole, this chapter aims to illustrate the nature of caregivers' relationships with
forgetful elders, and the way it reveals a tension with normative perspectives
of old age.

CAREGIVING CHALLENGES: "WE THINK ABOUT
THE FUTURE, AND HOW MUCH WORSE IT COULD GET"

Pablo and Vanessa's description of how their lives have become redefined by
caregiving—and their ambivalence toward it as they continued to remind me that
they were doing an act of charity—highlighted what is, perhaps, the practice's
most definitive feature. Caregiving is challenging. These challenges are every
day and increasingly difficult, placing emotional demands on caregivers that, in
turn, become another set of challenges toward how they attend to, empathize
or become frustrated with, and ultimately form new types of relationships with
elders. Pablo and Vanessa are challenged on a daily level by minor instances
like Maria's forgetting the comings and goings of people, and major ones like
jeopardizing the safety of their home. "There's been a big change. We don't have
a lot of freedom to go out as we used to [and] we're always pressured to return

as soon as possible," Pablo said, reflecting on their new role as caregivers. He further explained his sense of urgency: "She started to develop this bad habit where, if someone knocks on the door, she'll invite them in and she'll offer to sell anything within her reach. She'll sell anything for five or ten pesos."

Challenges like this represent the dimension of caregiving that is so often depicted in the literature, referred to through notions like "caregiver burden," what researchers call "the most compelling problem affecting caregivers" (Adelman et al., 2014, p. 1053; see also Drinka, Smith, & Drinka, 1987; Mahoney, Regan, Katona, & Livingston, 2005; Schulz & Williamson, 1991).[2] Yet in contrast to trends in gerontology, I do not view these challenges as "burdens" that caregivers are tasked to endure, but realities they elect to engage with because of their inherent meaning. And, whereas most research is framed in terms of the importance of early detection and techniques for caregivers to better cope, such attempts are inadequate so long as they overlook the ways this experience is constituted in caregivers' specific forms of relating to elders. Focus on the broader relationship puts into focus why smaller aggravations are so distressing to begin with; the challenges inherent in caregiving are, in part, representative of a larger change in the way caregivers come to see and relate to elders.[3]

This experience is not unique to Pablo and Vanessa's case but applicable to all the individuals I studied and, I suspect, definitive of care itself. As Kleinman (2011) says of his own experience caregiving for his wife, "caregiving . . . for dementia draws you into an enmeshed relationship. You begin to lose the self of your own self, because you're constantly entering [another's] space to do things for them." Much like Kleinman, each of the caregivers I studied described how their relationships with elders changed as a result of assuming new responsibilities. Analyzing what specific aspects of caregiving are challenging highlights this very point. The experiences caregivers perceive to be challenging are constituted by a combination of sincere love for elders and the way broader social outlooks constitute that affection. This latter factor is essential toward understanding what makes caregiving meaningful, how caregiving defines a new set of relations, and the way it comes to reshape the local meaning of aging.

In the majority of households, elders' tendency to wander was discussed as a challenge that caregivers faced on a daily level. Pablo and Vanessa took on their caregiving responsibilities after they noticed Maria begin to increasingly wander and get lost. "She wasn't able to remember where her sister's house was," Vanessa said. "And she would point at someone else's house, saying that it was her sister's house." This was one of the first symptoms Pablo and Vanessa noticed of Maria and they began to recognize that, as Maria increasingly became disoriented, she also jeopardized her safety. They worried about her boarding a bus and getting lost outside the community, or walking in rural parts of town with no one to help her should she get injured.

Concern about wandering was a similar topic of discussion among Sergio, Manuel, and Linda, the family highlighted in chapter 1, whose "tricky" father began to increasingly forget family names. They were still shaken up from the night Pedro got lost in Tijuana and described how, in Teotitlán, Pedro continues to try to leave home with little direction or purpose. Linda described how her husband is "always watching when people come to the house . . . so he can take advantage of an unlocked door." And Manuel further explained why his father's attempts to leave home are so concerning. Wandering is "what really worries us," he said. "It's very dangerous for him to get in a cab or a bus and get lost somewhere. And sometimes we get the worst thoughts. . . . He could get in a taxi and go somewhere, but the thing is he probably won't make it back. Just like what happened in Tijuana. That's why we always watch him, to make sure he doesn't go out, and that's the most concerning part of taking care of him." Indeed, wandering was a threat for the majority of caregivers and they often discussed how it changed the way they related to forgetful elders, making smaller responsibilities like locking doors and gates a larger concern to ensure elders' safety. In so doing, caregivers come to see elders as increasingly unable to make sound decisions and a liability to their own well-being. And this, they implicitly expressed, became a reality that led to a significant shift in how elders come to lose decision-making power.

In a similar vein, another common challenge cited by caregivers was that living with a forgetful elder is difficult because of the regularity of household conflicts.[4] While many caregivers stated that they did not view forgetfulness as problematic, they commonly described it as the cause for their frequent instances of fighting with elders.[5] For their part, Pablo and Vanessa described numerous instances of how hostility and conflicts have come to characterize their caregiving experience. When Pablo leaves home to weave for a merchant, Maria alleges that he is lying and instead has gone off to get drunk. This at first caused suspicion and fighting between Pablo and Vanessa, but they later learned to dismiss Maria's allegations. In other instances, Vanessa said that she and her children are often accused of stealing or intentionally hiding things from Maria. One particularly bitter argument involved Maria accusing Vanessa of stealing her clothes and deliberately conspiring to make her life difficult. Vanessa recalled their exchange: "She told me that I wasn't a good person . . . and I told her, 'I'm trying to take care of you the best I can. And I think I'm doing a good job. . . . What I have to eat, I share with you. And now you pay me back in this way?' " Vanessa eventually asked her father to intervene and to explain to Maria that she needed to control her anger. But their arguments persisted, and Vanessa eventually came to accept this as part of what her responsibilities now entail.

How Pablo and Vanessa came to regularly argue with Maria was also the center of meaning when they learned that Maria had Alzheimer's disease. When these outbursts first appeared two years ago, they thought that Maria's behavior was simply attributable to anger. "I didn't pay attention to [her anger] because I thought that was just her getting old," Vanessa said. "I thought that she was just being aggressive with us." They hoped that Maria would recover from mourning her husband and that her anger would subside, and, ultimately, that the household would return to a sense of normalcy. But they explained how Maria's being diagnosed with Alzheimer's disease upended these hopes. Pablo explained, "That caused us to worry more about her. Because we see her and we know and we understand that she has an illness. And so there is more to worry about, and we think about what's going to happen in the future. Because she could get worse. And we think about the future, and how much worse it could get." Indeed, learning that Maria's behavioral changes did not stem from anger, but from a recognized illness, significantly changed how Pablo and Vanessa understand their situation. Instead of time serving as a hopeful promise for improvement, it became a threat of the progression of symptoms to come. This ultimately changed how Pablo and Vanessa related to Maria: from having viewed her as a person whose anger was under her control and a meaningful expression of sadness, toward seeing her as a person whose anger was a symptom of dependency and need for care.[6]

As Pablo and Vanessa initially viewed Maria's anger as a personal attack, caregivers from other households noted how they argued with elders over seemingly insignificant topics. To consider a different household, arguments began to appear not long after Luis and Laura decided to move in with Laura's widowed mother because she appeared increasingly unable to remain safe while living alone as a widow. They described how minor accusations were representative of larger, more serious challenges. For example, Laura described how she was similarly blamed for misplacing her mother's possessions and, in general, felt that her mother was constantly provoking arguments. "Of course it affects me," Laura said, "Because she's always blaming me that I hide things from her."

And she's always sure that I'm the one that hides it from her. I don't know why she can't think to ask me in a polite manner where her purse is—because there's a way you can ask someone in a respectful way. Like, "Have you seen my bag, by any chance?" But what she does [is] she's always pointing her finger at me and is sure that I'm the one that took it. And I think that's something that always gets me angry. And we start arguing. And I have a lot of things to do instead of hiding her bags. So I don't have time to do that. And I tell her that, "I'm tired of you treating me this way." And this is an everyday problem.

The manner by which Laura conveys the relentlessness of her mother's accusations is telling. Laura's use of words and phrases like "always," "everyday," and "I'm tired" helps convey how these instances have come to be definitive of everyday life. Her mother's accusations make it difficult to do chores and, more distressing, Laura loses patience herself.

As a whole, these accusations highlight how caregiving is not a challenging job merely because of what occurs in the household, but also for the implications and larger changes that occur in the relationships caregivers share with elders. That is why the above caregivers do not experience accusations or elders' tendency to wander as distressing per se. Their distress comes from the way elders test their patience, increasingly show their confusion, and are subsequently seen in a different perspective. In a context where family cohesion and respect for elders is celebrated as part of local tradition—where elders are viewed through the ideal of the bengul—one could understand that these challenges are a signifier of larger social change. Household conflict and elders' tendency to wander are not merely challenging because they require caregivers to adapt to new domestic circumstances, but because they also invoke concerns about maintaining idealized notions of cohesion in context of contemporary life.

This point is perhaps best made through discussing another set of challenges—elders' incontinence and related dependencies regarding basic bodily functions. This is what some term "the dirty work of caregiving," described as one of the "most serious threats to caregivers' sense of self" (Jervis, 2001, p. 84). In the households I studied, these challenges further represent larger changes to how caregivers relate to elders. In their case, Pablo and Vanessa said that despite all of the challenges they faced throughout the day, bathing and helping Maria go to the toilet was most challenging. "One of the hardest things in taking care of her is to shower her," Vanessa said. "Because I have to take off all of her clothes, and I have to take out all of the clean clothes for her to use." Vanessa described how Maria is often confused about how to shower and change her clothes, but also that Maria occasionally is too weak to stand on her own and needs to be physically supported to be bathed.

This difficulty repeatedly came up during my research on Mario, Isabelle, and Graciela, the caregivers highlighted in the previous chapter. After his last stroke, Nicholas not only lost ability to walk and verbally communicate, but also became incontinent. In their communal courtyard, far from the street and far from earshot, Isabelle leaned in to whisper, "He can't do his necessities." And Mario clarified, "Now that he's in this state, we have to change his soiled pants—I have to change it. He's not able to go to the bathroom . . . and he does it at any time." Like Pablo and Vanessa, Mario's statement points to the harsh reality that his father cannot control his bowels and must be helped in the most basic of ways. It is difficult for Mario to acknowledge, and embarrassing for Isabelle, who describes their work in a whisper that communicates her self-consciousness. Indeed, Nicholas has not only lost symbolic authority as bengul, he appears to have lost command of his own body. In acknowledging this reality, Mario and Isabelle intimate shame. They feed off each other's words, appearing taciturn and reluctant. They sense that the challenges they face are unusual and difficult for others to imagine, and that their experience with Nicholas stands in contrast to the way neighbors view elders in the community.

Facing the reality of incontinence is an additional instance of how caregivers are challenged to take on greater responsibility for elders' well-being. It touches on what Kleinman (2011) terms "caregiving enmeshment," when "your own subjectivity becomes part of their subjectivity [and] their subjectivity is part of you." The boundary that formerly separated Mario from his father becomes blurred, leading to greater fusion between caregivers and elders. Yet enmeshment and dependency do not signify the same thing across time and space. In contrast to U.S. settings, where self-sufficiency is so prioritized, in Teotitlán enmeshment invokes local values regarding how elders have the last word and how they are normatively given respect. In Teotitlán all family members are considered dependent on one another, jointly contributing to the household and part of the larger family cohesion. Here, in contrast, the dependency occasioned by not being able to manage human necessities is an illustration of elders' gradual loss of authority in the home.

Though so many caregivers cited arguments, wandering, and attending to human necessities as being central to what made their experiences challenging, this alone does not explain why meeting with caregivers was so laden with emotion—how I encountered so many caregivers who spoke through tears. Death looms. These elders, who are increasingly dependent on caregivers, are expected to pass away. Indeed, elders' increasing dependence is a daily reminder that death and dying is a reality that families must face.

This is how I understand Carlos, the husband who cared for his diabetic wife with her finger amputation and severe Alzheimer's. At one point, Carlos described how his life has been affected by caring for his wife:

> It was difficult. Because we always worked together. And since we were in the rug business, she's the one that helped me to wash and dye the yarn. So we did everything together. But when she started to forget, it was very difficult for me. Because there was no one else that could help me. . . . It's difficult in many ways. For everything and in everything.

Carlos's statement provides insight on gender labor divisions, but here I want to focus on the more encompassing point about how he and his wife formed a partnership to mutually provide and care for each other. The progressive dissolution of their partnership is what Carlos is forced to recognize. It is a challenge centered on the ongoing losses they have endured together, and the final one he anticipates witnessing without her. It is about feeling limited toward the way domestic responsibilities have been allotted, and also because he is forced to imagine a life without his wife, a life in which he anticipates being socially unmoored. Carlos describes this in curious but heartfelt terms—"for everything and in everything"—that is, he experiences it for every reason, and during every moment. This challenge is not only unique to Carlos, but was discussed among all caregivers as they recognize that forgetfulness and dependency are representative of the aging process itself. It is a challenge that appears to eclipse other challenges, despite how subtle it is and how harsh others may immediately prove.

Though I apply greater focus on local ideas about death and dying in the following chapter, here I want to briefly address how the challenge of anticipating loss is also constituted within a specific cultural landscape. In Oaxaca, death is not considered a sudden event that comes to separate the living from the dead, but rather an ongoing social process that is part of everyday life experience.[7] In her study of Oaxacan death customs, Norget (2006) describes how everyday life is structured by concerns to treat deceased family members properly. She writes, in Oaxaca "it is the responsibility of the living to ensure the well-being of the dead; not to do so puts the whole community in danger" (p. 17; see also Royce, 2011). How one anticipates and provides for another's death carries immense weight in the local consciousness. People are not only expected to respect elders, but also provide a space to allow them to die in peace—and it is believed that if this space is not provided, the deceased will return to haunt the living. This perspective adds an additional challenge for caregivers. It highlights how simultaneously experiencing conflict and losing traditional forms of respect for elders create tension and, more generally, how caregiving challenges are again woven in a broader cultural fabric.

As a whole, my purpose in enumerating caregiving challenges is, first, to illustrate the daily experiences of caregiving and, second, to highlight how these experiences lead to new ways of perceiving elders. From intra-family fighting, wandering, meeting basic human necessities, and recognizing the reality of death, the challenges that caregivers face alter how elders are viewed and positioned within the household. While these challenges might be similar in other households in different cultural settings, their meaning and experience is specific to life in Teotitlán. They are constituted within broader social values, revealing a tension between the ideal of old age and family cohesion, and the reality of how these notions are negotiated in everyday caregiving experience.

ROLE REVERSAL: "WE WILL
CONSIDER HER MORE LIKE A CHILD"

Although Pablo and Vanessa said that they were not aware of any other elders with similar symptoms of forgetfulness in Teotitlán, Vanessa recalled a neighbor she knew during her childhood. This elder was known to forget and wander aimlessly through the community. Vanessa remembers how the elder used to throw rocks at people and hit walls, out of anger, often with a broomstick. The elder had no family to take care of her and eventually died in Oaxaca City. "At that time we were very young, and my dad used to say that she was possessed by a witch," Vanessa recalled. And she added, "I wonder to myself whether [what's happening to Maria] was what happened to that person." Yet while Vanessa's childhood memory shows it is easy to dismiss behavioral disturbances of a stranger as an instance of craziness or possession, her experience with Maria demonstrates it is more difficult to apply this perspective for those more intimately involved in the provision of care. Indeed, Pablo and Vanessa did not believe Maria was crazy or possessed by a witch, but the challenges they encountered did cause them to see her differently. They described how Maria has "completely changed" and how her frequent provocations have shifted the way they relate to her. At one point, Pablo reflected how the gradual appearance of Maria's anger led to a significant shift. "In the beginning, I told [Vanessa and my children] that she is no longer an adult. We will consider her more like a child. She would be doing this and that, or pulling this and that, or moving our things around. Her mentality is no longer the mentality of a healthy person. Compared to us, who think before we act, she does everything she's *not* supposed to do."

Much like Pablo and Vanessa have come to see Maria like a child, I found the same perspective endorsed among the majority of other caregivers, indicative of how caregivers come to form a different type of relationship with elders. Though comparing elders to children may appear to belittle elders, attentiveness to broader social dynamics highlights how it can serve a positive function that mitigates the challenges presented above.[8] It implicitly invokes a perspective about limited accountability and, specifically, how children are perceived to lack awareness of the world and lack basic understanding of their actions.[9] But by the same token, comparing elders to children leads to a different relationship that is premised on recognizing elders' dependency and vulnerability. This further highlights the discrepancy between how elders are idealized with authority and the reality that caregivers encounter at home.

In many Western settings, "role reversal" is a common description that describes the comparison of dependent elders to immature children. This idea points to the change that occurs when spouses, adult children, grandchildren, and other relatives become "parents" to elders who are no longer able to support themselves. Originally described in an article written by Arthur Rautman (1962), the concept points to how the perceived autonomy that once distinguished parents from their children slowly becomes blurred and eventually "reversed" in the aging process.[10] Though dated, role reversal continues to be featured in much of contemporary literature on caregiving and has become a taken-for-granted description. For example, in *The 36 Hour Day* (2011), what many consider the most useful handbook on dementia caregiving, Mace and Rabins distinguish between responsibilities and roles (pp. 195–99).[11] Responsibilities are the jobs assigned to family members; they may or may not change, and their inherent malleability shows how they are not determinative of the way the individual is viewed. By contrast, roles are the ways people are seen and understood within the family. Individuals carry specific roles that are created and solidified by family interaction. Whereas cooking dinner is a responsibility, being a voice of authority is a role. The point is that role changes are more difficult to accept and adjust to—which explains why, to return to Pablo's statements about Maria acting like a child, role changes are so important to understand. Such perspectives signal a fundamental shift in identity, reconfiguring who a caregiver is in relation to how a forgetful elder is now seen.

Pablo and Vanessa were far from the only caregivers to describe elders as children, and it is telling that so many others did as well.[12] For some caregivers, viewing elders as children is a way to cope with their anticipation of an elder's death. This was the case for Francisca, a caregiver in her early sixties, and her 30-year-old daughter, Dominga. Together they cared for Antonio, Francisca's brother, an elder in his early eighties who had a severe series of strokes, combined with the recent onset seizures. Over the course of eight years, Antonio has increasingly become dependent on Francisca and Dominga's care. At the time I met them, Antonio had just had a stroke that now impaired his ability to walk. Antonio's seizures were also becoming more severe and frequent; he lost consciousness almost weekly and, in combination with his stroke history, developed significant memory loss. He had difficulty sustaining conversation and continually expressed confusion about daily life. He had also begun to hallucinate being attacked by animals and has started to yell in a sense of panic. Francisca and Dominga described feeling helpless in the face of the growing severity of Antonio's condition, and said that they were certain he would soon pass away. In this context, Dominga said, "I can't say that I look at him in the same way I used to look at him. I look at him now as a kid. Like if he was a person that is there, but not there. Am I making sense? That's the way we look at him. We only look at a body. But he is not there." Like other caregivers, Dominga has begun to look at Antonio like a child but here, she expresses how this perspective is a way to begin recognizing his anticipated death. She distinguishes between body and soul; his soul has progressively departed, while his body remains alive.[13] Despite his not being dead, Dominga shows how this perspective orients her to see Antonio as if he already were. Viewing him as a child helps prepare Dominga for the reality she knows will soon come.

While Dominga's case illustrates how comparing elders to children helps manage distress in anticipating an elder's death, throughout my research I came across numerous other instances where caregivers highlighted how this perspective also furnishes a means to accept and cope with the challenges they

encountered on a daily basis. For example, as Juanita cared for her husband
through remedies that she learned in her practice as a *curandera*, she talked
about how she continues to feel challenged by her husband's inability to bathe
or go to the restroom by himself. In the process of explaining the challenges
she faced, Juanita described her husband in a language strikingly similar to
Pablo and Vanessa.

> When he needs to go to the bathroom, he isn't able to do it by
> himself. . . . And the same thing happens when he needs to bathe.
> We have to get him ready, get his water ready, *just like a child*. We
> have to have his clothes ready, his towel, and we have to monitor
> him while showering so he doesn't wet his towel or clothes. And
> we also have to watch when he dresses, especially when he puts his
> shoes on, because he tends to put them on wrong. (Emphasis added.)

As she would ensure that children bathe properly, Juanita states that she takes the
same precautions with her husband. Caregiving, she suggests, is like parenting.
Juanita is not only describing the presence of new responsibilities associated with
parenting; she is saying that she has, in a metaphorical sense, become a parent.
Juanita's responsibilities are symbolic of a new way of relating to her husband,
a reminder that they cannot maintain the same relationship they shared prior.

Similarly, when Sergio, Manuel, and Linda discussed how their father got
lost in Tijuana and has come to increasingly forget their names, they also talked
about how Pedro has become "tricky" in his attempts to leave home and misplace
objects. Together, they reflected on how these behaviors have shifted their
perspective of him.

MANUEL: Well, right now I see him more like a child rather than my dad.
SERGIO: Me too. I see him as a child. Because sometimes he gets me pretty
angry. Because sometimes I tell him to do something very gently, but
he just doesn't do it.
LINDA: A few days ago we were preparing *maize* [taking corn off the husk]
and I got distracted just for a second. [Then] I realized he was throwing
the husks at me. And later he just walked on the corn. And also started
mixing the *maize*, the good ones with the bad ones.
SERGIO: And just like I said earlier, he asked me, "Who's my dad?" But I
didn't tell him anything. So I don't pay much attention to him, since I
know that he doesn't remember. So I just try to bear with him, because
I can't argue with him. Even though there's often so much friction.

Once again, this household described their perspective of Pedro as a child. They reason that this perspective is justified by how Pedro provokes arguments and is tricky, and they proceed to express how viewing him as a child helps them see him as a different, less accountable member of the family. Yes, he is nominally their father or husband, but his behavior is unrecognizable, and he appears to be a different person—a child.

These statements are just a sample of what nearly all caregivers expressed.[14] Given the variability across households I studied, the differing levels of severity caregivers noted, and the divergent opinions among members within the same households, it is telling how prevalent this perspective was. Yet despite how often role reversal was discussed during interviews—and how prevalent it is in U.S. caregiving literature—geriatric researchers argue against its continued use in describing caregiving relations. Their critique stands on two grounds. First, they argue that role reversal is an inaccurate way to describe the caregiving relationship; it equates caregiving with parenting when, in fact, adult children know that the recipients of their care—their parents—are not children at all. As Mildred Seltzer (1990) writes, "children remain children to their parents all their lives" (p. 9). Along this line of reasoning, role reversal is inaccurate because it does not account for the meaning of caregiving: caring for a dependent elder presages increasing dependency, whereas with children one anticipates increasing independence. Second, and more importantly, researchers also argue that role reversal is destructive to the caregiving relationship. It maintains ageist assumptions by depreciating elders as children, foreclosing respect, and denying the possibility of reciprocated familial relationships (Brody, 1990). Yet caregivers know that elders are not actually children, and they also do not negate that elders remain their husbands, wives, fathers, mothers, and so forth. For this reason, I make a distinction between what some researchers call "classic role reversal" and what I term metaphorical role reversal, a perspective that likens elders to children, but does not posit that they have actually become children (see Hargrave and Anderson, 2013, pp. 17–18). This latter position is a metaphor in Lakoff and Johnson's (1980) use of the term, a means to orient oneself to a new situation by reference to a more familiar one.

Viewing role reversal metaphorically helps us appreciate how caregivers' comments about elders being like children are an act of construction—once again, constructed from surrounding discourse and constructive of the world. In part, caregivers compare elders to children because of their own parenting experiences. Like Pablo and Vanessa have three young children, many other caregivers were also in what gerontologists call the "sandwich generation," responsible for caring not only for dependent elders but also for dependent children (Brody, 1985; Miller, 1981). Caregivers know what caring for children is like, and thus compare their work with elders to this. But talk about elders as being like children is also constructive—it fosters a type of relationship with elders that would be different without such talk. As Pablo expressed, through explicitly deciding to view Maria like a child, he and his family are able to understand and relate to changes that stand at odds with how Maria is expected to behave. Comparing elders to children can be understood as an attempt to work through the tension between how old age is idealized and the reality caregivers encounter.

CAREGIVING STRATEGIES: "PLEASE DO NOT ACT LIKE THAT, BECAUSE YOU CAN GET WORSE"

A few days before I met them, Pablo and Vanessa noticed a peculiar change in Maria's behavior. In contrast to how they were accustomed to Maria's accusations that they or their children stole things, Maria began to claim that she saw a young girl enter her room to rob her belongings. At first, Maria said she saw the girl remove and steal the fabric she used to braid her hair. Then she saw her run off another time with the TV remote. Pablo and Vanessa are certain that no girl has visited their home, and the frequency Maria began to claim to see the girl made them conclude that she does not, in fact, exist. Yet instead of contesting Maria, they reasoned it would be best to empathize with her frustration and to help find her lost belongings. "I try to talk to her in a kind way," Vanessa said of her new approach. "And I tell her, 'Are you looking for your things?' And she'll respond, 'Yes, that girl took it.' And then I tell her, 'Don't be upset,' and I hold her hand and help her look for it." Vanessa's attempts to help calm Maria are expressive of the broader set of practices that make up caregiving. Together, they are representative of caregivers' attempts to live with and morally respond to the challenges they face on a daily level.

"Care seeks to lighten what is heavy, and even if it fails it keeps on trying," write Mol, Moser, and Pols (2010, p. 14). Indeed, all of the caregivers in this study exemplified this perspective, and discussed how they practiced the type of "persistent tinkering" described by Mol and colleagues—care that adapts to the ever-changing challenges inherent to their experience (p. 14). Whereas in previous pages I explored how challenges and perspectives of elders as children reconstitute how caregivers view elders, in this final section I explore the specific strategies that come to behaviorally define the caregiving relationship. By "strategies" I mean the interventions, techniques, and other forms of action taken by caregivers to concretely care for elders and address the challenges they face. Following Wilkinson and Kleinman (2016), this approach views caregiving as a *phronesis* (a form of "practical wisdom") that does not involve abstract reasoning about how to care for elders, but concrete day-to-day adjustment—"tinkering"—to live optimally in the presence of change (p. 163). Enumerating these daily strategies helps provide a more comprehensive picture of caregiving, and also helps shed greater light on how it regenerates caregivers' relationships with elders. Insofar as forgetful elders are compared to children, caregivers' strategies demonstrate how this alternative vision is concretized in attempt to maintain values concerning family and household cohesion.

In light of Vanessa's response to Maria's hallucinations, she and Pablo have developed a broader strategy to be patient and appease her. They explained how they learned that they would not be successful directly contesting Maria when she accused people of stealing her objects. Instead, they strategized to agree with Maria and, in the process, try to help her reestablish a sense of security at home. Pablo said, "More than anything, we try to help her find whatever she's looking for in any given moment. That way she calms down quicker, because if we don't pay attention to it she gets worse." Later, he further explained how he and Vanessa came to agree on this approach:

> Well, what we try to do is agree with her [whenever she accuses us]. Just like we said, if she's arguing about something, we'll always agree with her. I'm the one that's always telling [Vanessa] to agree with whatever she says, since she's the one that takes care of her most of the time. Also because [Vanessa] gets stressed very quickly. With me, I try to calm down first and agree to anything she's saying. And when I agree with her she calms down a lot quicker. . . . So I often tell [Vanessa] to agree with whatever she says—after all, to agree doesn't mean that everything's going to change with her. Or that we're actually taking her stuff. . . . That's the way we try to make it easier.

Viewing Maria's behavior as resembling a child helps Pablo and Vanessa maintain their strategy. They appease and agree with Maria when she accuses people of stealing her belongings, try to avoid arguments about the facts that they know prove her wrong, and in the process try to ameliorate her distress. This helps illustrate how Pablo and Vanessa relate to Maria by privately (but not verbally) dismissing the validity of her accusations, but it also provides insight into their own relationship as caregivers. Aside from Pablo suggesting to Vanessa about how to optimally deal with Maria (which in itself is further expressive of local gender dynamics), this shows how they attempt to reestablish domestic harmony in the presence of discord. Among themselves they recognize a reality that they abstain from mentioning to Maria so as not to further provoke her. Ultimately, they reason that contesting the truth of Maria's accusations does not matter as much trying to pacify her and reestablish peace in their home.

Whereas Pablo's statements expressed that being patient with elders is a means to establish peace at home, caregivers also explained that this strategy is central toward providing the care they know elders need. This was implicit in Pablo's remarks, but more directly discussed at other moments as well. Vanessa said that she tries to be calm and agreeable when Maria is agitated because she worries that Maria's anger will worsen her condition. This is an implicit reference to her etiological understanding of the cause of Maria's condition. In contrast to U.S. settings, where repression of anger is viewed to be dangerous, researchers have long noted the inverse in Mexico—that expression of anger is perceived to be sickness-producing (Finkler, 1997, p. 1148; Hunt, 1992, p. 310; Wentzell, 2013, p. 93). Drawing on this understanding, Vanessa described how she practices patience when she is accused of stealing Maria's possessions.

> I try to calm her down and I tell her that we'll go look for it. And when I find it I tell her "Look it's here," and I show it to her. . . . That's why I tell her, "Please do not act like that, because you can get worse, and if that happens, who else is going to take care of you?" . . . She forgets her stuff and what I do to calm her down. I try to hold her hands, and sit with her, and then when I think she's better, I go back to work to resume weaving.

Here Vanessa provides greater context to how she is patient with Maria, and why she views it as central to providing good care. Her words are calm, understanding, and mollifying. She does not want to further agitate Maria and even tries to reason with her, despite knowing that reason is not what will engage her. In the process of explaining this strategy, we get a perspective of why calming elders is important. It helps manage elders' distress and prevent their condition from worsening. As such, patience is not only a means to maintain peace at home, but also a strategy to attend to elders' needs. But regardless of which rationale they focus on, patience redefines how Vanessa engages with

Maria and the nature of their relationship. Like a child, Maria is not someone whose thoughts and opinions are respected without question, but someone whose distress must be pacified.

This change in how caregivers relate to elders is perhaps more evident in other strategies. Like so many others, Pablo and Vanessa talked about how Maria's tendency to wander was problematic and how they strategized to ensure her safety by monitoring and confining her. While Vanessa spent most of her time at home weaving, she occasionally ran errands that left Maria unattended. Vanessa explained, "Sometimes there are places that both of us have to go. I can't go freely because I feel pressure to return as soon as possible. Because I don't know where she is, what she might be doing [at home]. . . . So I tell [Pedro] that we should hurry to get back home. And so I worry a lot for her." Though they recognized it was dangerous to allow Maria to rummage through the home and explore objects in places like the kitchen, where she could start a fire, they reasoned that locking her at home was a better alternative than allowing her to wander in the streets.

This strategy was discussed by the majority of caregivers whose elders were mobile, and most salient among Sergio, Manuel, and Linda, as they were still shaken from when Pedro was lost in Tijuana. Similar to Vanessa, at one point Sergio said, "I think that it's easier—or what makes things less stressful—is when we lock him up. Even though when we lock him up he touches everything that's in the room . . . and touches everything he knows he's not supposed to. But at least he's safe there, and I know where he is." There is an obvious simplicity to this strategy: as caregiving is challenging because elders are prone to wander, one solution is to confine them to one place. It helps ensure elders' safety and mollify caregivers' concerns. But also implicit in this strategy is the perspective that elders put their own safety in jeopardy. Once again, this stands in further contrast between the reality caregivers must acknowledge of forgetful elders and the respect that families are normatively expected to give.

Whereas the above perspectives illustrate how caregivers' strategies put in tension the ideal of the elder as bengul, other strategies to engage elders through conversation and activity further testify to changes in caregivers' relationships with elders. For example, Pablo and Vanessa described why they decided to engage Maria through assigning her household chores. At one point Pablo explained, "She's not able to cook anymore. But there are a few things that she still can do. So, to avoid any fights and arguments, we let her do [the dishes]. But before [Vanessa] uses any of them, she washes them because Maria doesn't do it properly." Pablo and Vanessa described how giving Maria household chores makes her feel useful and further prevents arguments. They explained that keeping Maria active and engaging her in domestic life gives her a sense of purpose at home and, by so doing, distracts her from thinking too much about her deceased husband.

Other caregivers described similar strategies to keep elders engaged. After they began to notice her becoming increasingly forgetful, Luis and Laura described their efforts to keep Laura's mother occupied. Their explanation of this strategy provides further rationale into why caregivers view mental and physical activity as important to elders' well-being. Laura explained:

> A few days ago I tried to talk to her. I asked her if there was something going on with her. "You should find something to do at home like sweeping the house, or doing some chores. That's what I think. I might be wrong." But what does she do when she's home? All she does is sit down and that's it; she sits all day long. And of course that makes her think too much. And instead, if she were to keep herself busy, she would be distracted. After all, every day we have something to do here, especially women's chores . . . there are dishes to wash . . . or she could sweep the house, and get things ready so that when I get back from the market we could eat breakfast. And she could even prepare chocolate or salsa. But instead, she just remains mad at us.

Laura's words similarly demonstrate how she views activity as a means to provide care she knows her mother needs. She sees her mother's forgetfulness and anger as related to her thinking too much and, as a result, Laura tries to get her mother to be active and distracted. But in the process, Laura develops another reason to argue with her mother. She gets frustrated that her mother does not listen to her advice or contribute to household chores. She gets frustrated that her mother thinks too much. And, for her part, Laura's mother responds in anger that she is being told what to do. This dynamic helps further illustrate the role change in caregiving households. In encouraging elders to be active and not get worse, caregivers assume an assertive stance that is at odds with how elders are normatively treated. This accounts for the frustration Laura experiences, and the anger her mother displays in response.

Attempting to engage and converse with elders was also a strategy for caregivers when they noticed elders become withdrawn from more than just domestic chores. This was implicit in Pablo and Vanessa's rationale for engaging with Maria when she appeared to think too much about her husband, but it was also stated among other caregivers who dealt with more severe forms of dementia. With Cynthia's development of Alzheimer's, and well after her finger amputation, which her family understood to be the cause of her thinking too much, Carlos and his son, Francisco, discussed how they continually tried to include and engage Cynthia in the family's social happenings. Francisco described their strategy:

> We try to include her in conversation, we try to start speaking with her, regardless of her difficulties responding. And we try to get her out. . . . For example, when we all get together, we invite her to join us, so she's able to participate with us. And we see the change—she becomes more content. . . . She likes it. Because when she's alone that's when she seems more depressed. But when we're all together and she hears us talking and she participates.

Francisco's words are significant when considering the severity of his mother's "complete" forgetfulness. She can hardly speak, walk, and carry out other basic functions. Still, Carlos and Francisco say they seek Cynthia's participation and note positive reactions. She laughs and even seems to convey a basic sense of understanding of the social life around her. She appears less depressed and thus less prone to further decline. In this way, engaging Cynthia is not only a way to provide her the care she needs, but is also a way to meet caregivers' needs as well—to foster a sense of family cohesion in the presence of progressive loss.

In reviewing these common strategies, we gain an appreciation for the practices that make up caregiving on a daily basis. These strategies are simultaneously aimed to give elders the care that they need, while they also function to provide family and household cohesion in an environment where cohesion is called into question. Caregivers show how they draw on multiple strategies, continually "tinkering" them to find solutions that work. They simultaneously seek to minimize disruptions to household unity, ensure that elders' needs are met, and take related action to prevent future decline. Each strategy draws on local values about what the good life amounts to, but each also illustrates how the same values are put in tension through caregiving practice. Caregivers not only compare elders to children, but concretely change the ways they engage with them. In the process, the relationship they share with elders is reconstituted through the practice of giving and receiving care.

~

This chapter has advanced three interrelated points on the local experience of caregiving. First, in describing caregiving challenges, the chapter demonstrates how caregivers experience forgetful elders as a challenge to maintaining a sense of family and household cohesion, and how this experience acknowledges fundamental changes to the relationship they share. Second, these challenges culminate in a different way of seeing elders—one that compares them to children, in contrast to the authority they are traditionally prescribed. While this perspective helps foster cohesion and helps caregivers better cope with the challenges they face, it also redefines what growing old means in the context of forgetfulness and related dependencies. Third, the chapter reviews caregiving strategies to depict how caregiving is practiced on a daily basis. It illustrates how caregivers strive to maintain local values, but simultaneously redefine the way they relate to elders. As a whole, this chapter puts in focus a tension between the ideal of the elder as bengul—as figure of authority and wisdom—and the reality of the ways forgetful elders are viewed through everyday caregiving experience.

This tension stands at the center of what caregivers find meaningful in attending to forgetful elders, and how they experience difficulty as they encounter the progressive losses associated with dementia. The tension also illustrates the discrepancy between the reality caregivers face on a daily basis and the contrastive norms they are held accountable to in the broader community. "People used to say that when elders forget they are crazy people," Pablo said reflecting on the difference between his experience as caregiver and the way he knows his efforts are misunderstood by the larger community. "They don't see things the way we do. That's why I personally think this is a very big experience. And whenever someone might need advice I'll be able to give it to them. I'll be able to say what taking care of an elder is like. This is pretty much like going to school." Much like going to school, Pablo states that caregiving has taught him a reality about aging that stands in contrast to how it is depicted by the broader community. He has learned about how aging could involve a form of decline that challenges the social authority old age is so often indexed to. And he has learned about how maintaining some aspects of local tradition might put others in question. In the process, Pablo has developed life experiences that set him apart from neighbors. Much like elders are known for the advice they give, Pablo says he is now able to offer his own. Caregiving has rendered him into a new figure of authority—a *bingul*—a younger person who is mature and distinguished by his own accumulated wisdom as caregiver. He will be able to speak about the importance and the challenges of caring for dependent elders, about the inherent tension of upholding local values in the wake of social change, and the experience of bringing family together in moments when it feels most questioned.

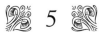

5

Relationships With the Community

SHARED VALUES, MISUNDERSTANDINGS, AND THE SECOND FORGOTTEN SUBJECT

Sophia shared photographs that she had kept in a *Costco 1 Hour Photo* envelope. I agreed that her year-old grandson was beyond charming and, as we looked at the collection one-by-one, she explained how these images helped bridge distance to feel closer to her family. Three of Sophia's five adult children live in California. They are all married, with their own children. The remaining two daughters live in Teotitlán, but in their own homes with their husbands' families. So, Sophia lives alone and is the sole caregiver for Vicente, her 77-year-old husband recovering from a series of strokes. She said that living apart from her family has been difficult, but her children have cobbled together financial resources to support them. "We don't lack anything," she said, and further described how her children send remittances, clothes, and other forms of support.

Alex and I met Sophia in a home reminiscent of southern California suburbia—two-storied and beige-plastered, expansive rooms and bright-white painted walls—without question the most costly home I had encountered during my fieldwork. Vicente had formerly owned a local business selling baked goods, but the majority of their wealth came from remittances sent from California. When we first approached the house, walking up a dirt road in the fringes of the community, Vicente was in the front yard pulling weeds from a garden, and

Sophia greeted us while taking a break from mopping the kitchen tile floors. The house certainly conveyed prestige, but it also felt empty inside. Our voices were followed by a slight echo. And we sat on new plastic chairs next to an adjacent folding table in an otherwise unfurnished living room. Sophia explained how she and Vicente had their own home down the street, but her daughter and son-in-law had built this residence while living in California. Sophia and Vicente moved in three years ago to look after it.

At 65 years old, Sophia was unique in being the only caregiver I encountered alone, without other family members present. Her experience was laden with loneliness. "I'm the only one that takes care of him," Sophia said, "We're the only two that live here." She described the challenges of compensating for her children's decision to migrate and responding to what researchers term the "care slot," the meaningful absence of migrant family members who would otherwise distribute caregiving responsibilities among the larger family unit (Leinaweaver, 2010; Parreñas, 2015; Scott, 2012; Yarris, 2017). Sophia described this in expressive, heartfelt terms and, at times, showed difficulty speaking. "I'm scared," she said expressing herself through tears. "I'm scared because if he dies, I will be alone."

Though Sophia was unique in living apart from other family members, her fear of being alone and her struggle responding to family absences was common to some degree among all caregivers I studied. This touches on what Holly Worthen (2012) aptly calls "the presence of absence." Every household had at least one member working and living abroad, leading to a felt internal tension about how to distribute caregiving responsibilities while continuing to pursue their lives in the broader community.

In this chapter I explore the suffering inherent to caregiving and how it is expressive of caregivers' social lives in the broader community. Though it may seem exaggerated to refer to caregiving experience as an instance of suffering, I deliberately choose this term to highlight how it involves a certain type of difficulty—a suffering—that is social in nature. As an extension of the approach taken in the previous chapter, what follows is an analysis of suffering as one element of subjectivity that is constituted by the broader social world. According to research on social suffering, even an experience as basic as pain is not just a physiological response to a physical stressor, but inextricable to the social world that gives rise to it—economic parameters, political regimes, cultural values, and more; one could not make sense of pain without attending to these social realms. In this perspective, traditional dichotomies like "individual" and "collective" collapse and illustrate how suffering is at once collective *and* individual (see Das et al., 2000; Das et al., 2001; Holmes, 2013; Kleinman et al., 1997; Wilkinson & Kleinman, 2016). Critics argue against this approach for the way it tends to convey suffering as something that is universal. We all experience suffering, so the approach might implicitly suggest one can know what another's suffering is about and how to respond to it. Yet this comes at the expense of attending to the way suffering varies, dependent on the way it is culturally constituted (Robbins, 2013; see also Fassin, 2012). However much this might be fair criticism, I continue to engage with literature on social suffering precisely because suffering appeared so central toward understanding the caregivers I studied. In Sophia's case, the suffering she described was laden in nearly all her descriptions of care. Hers was a suffering that was at once personal and located within a broader social world where adult children migrate to pursue economic opportunity, and remaining family members are faced with the challenge of how to maintain local values in a setting where those values are questioned and renegotiated. Suffering is concomitant with the pursuit of these values, and attending to Sophia's suffering does not need to overlook how it is uniquely constituted by these broader social circumstances.

While one of her daughters initially offered to help care for Vicente, Sophia declined the offer for fear of upsetting him. Vicente denied being ill and Sophia did not want to contradict his perspective. Sophia explained that she had reason to be fearful. "He was a very angry person, a very angry person," Sophia said to emphasize her husband's character prior to his strokes. "When he was healthy, if someone was talking while we were eating, he would get mad. And he would tell them that if they're going to talk, they should talk outside." Vicente was high-tempered toward his entire family, and Sophia said she was regularly subject to verbal and physical abuse. This complicated how Sophia felt about her husband's current disability: at once a relief from his abuse, anticipating his death was also a threat toward her sense of security. "When he was healthy I was always scared of him. I was scared whenever he came back home. . . . But now, no. Now, instead of me feeling free from that oppression, I feel that if he were to die, I don't think I would be able to overcome it." Sophia simultaneously worried about losing her husband, and feared the abuse she would be subject to, were he to recover. This only intensified her loneliness.

Sophia's story integrates many themes from previous chapters and further helps situate her suffering. After a doctor diagnosed Vicente as having a stroke one year ago, Sophia noted periods of improvement, followed by abrupt declines. Sophia found the physician's explanation useful to account for these changes. "He said that a vein in his head clots and it un-clots. . . . When it clots, that's when the forgetting starts. And when it un-clots, that's when he starts to remember." Though he seemed to recover and continued to take prescribed medications, Vicente continued to have additional strokes. Their frequency and impact seemed to indicate he was progressively getting worse. Four months ago, after his last stroke, Sophia described Vicente's alarming condition:

> At that time, he was like only a living body [Zapotec original: *benn̄*, in this context literally "a person who is a stranger"]. He wouldn't say anything, and even if he saw me crying, he wouldn't care. For instance, I started crying when I saw him in that state—but he wouldn't say a thing. He wouldn't even ask what was wrong with me. Because when he was in good health, when he saw me crying, he would get mad. And he would say to me, "Oh you're going to start again, you cursed woman." But [after this last stroke], even when I cried, he just stared at me.

Sophia further described these alarming changes. She told of him being stuck at home, and worried about him wandering or injuring himself. "He completely forgot everything," she said, and then further reflected on how being the only person who cared for Vicente made her life difficult. "I didn't go out anymore. I didn't even go to the market."

Though Sophia described Vicente's condition as owing to brain clotting, she also speculated about other causes. "Well, the way I see it, it was probably because he was very mean. And now he is actually thinking about what he did when he was younger. . . . And I believe that he's regretting everything, and that's why he's forgetting." She appealed to notions about Vicente thinking too much as causing his forgetfulness, but also speculated that he might have also lost his soul once after being scared by a snake while tending to cattle. In this way, Sophia supplemented the medical treatment that Vicente was given by taking him to the site where he was thought to have lost his soul. Sophia described her efforts:

> I took water, flowers, and food for us to eat there. I also took a blanket so he could sleep there . . . so he could get his soul back. . . . And I sat next to him. I took bread, and sprinkled it all around, just like a *curandera* does. So I did that, and he fell asleep there. I also took holy water and a bamboo reed to use to call his name [and entice his soul to return].

Vicente gradually improved through the combined course of these efforts. "I
think the doctor's medication is doing a good job because he's getting better,"
Sophia said. But she added that her attempts to keep Vicente busy and reestablish
a sense of equilibrium must have helped as well. Sophia tried to keep him active
and avoid thinking too much, and provided detail about how she encouraged
Vicente to be active in the garden:

> I ask him to help me to weed the garden, and that, I think, helps him
> to stop thinking too much. That's why I keep him busy. I start doing
> things first, and then I ask him to help me. And now he's progressing.
> He's doing it the way he's supposed to. Because before, he used to do
> it like a kid that just plays around. He would just scratch the dirt. He
> didn't understand what he was doing. But now he understands. . . .
> Now he's able to weed the way he's supposed to.

Vicente has improved in other ways, too. He can now dress and take care of other
basic functions, like to go the bathroom. And, much to Sophia's relief so she can
get out of the house, Vicente has started driving again—though he continues to
need her help navigating because he gets lost or forgets where they are going.

Yet Sophia worried these gains were temporary and that Vicente's condition
will likely worsen. These concerns further capture reasons for why Sophia
suffers. She explained how she has dedicated herself to Vicente's recovery
because she does not want to have regrets that she could have done more:

> Now that he is sick, I try to take care of him the best I can. And
> my brother always tells me that I should have patience and to take
> care of him the best I can. Because if he ever passes away, I will
> not regret anything. . . . I will not treat him bad, or miss a meal
> for him. To the contrary, I'll provide everything for him. And my
> brother often reminds me that the time for him has come, and no
> one knows what day it will be. "It could be any day now," he says,
> "so you should take care of him so you will not regret that you
> neglected something. And forget about everything he did to you.
> In the end, he's your husband."

These are the norms that help structure and justify Sophia's efforts, but they
also lead to the inherent tension Sophia experiences. Devoting herself to care
for Vicente helps fulfill expectations for how she ought to support her husband,
but this also renders her isolated from engaging with and feeling understood by

people outside her home. She is lonely. Indeed, Sophia's reasons for devoting herself are central to what makes caregiving meaningful but, in addition to the loss she anticipates, they also constitute so much of her suffering.

In what follows, I continue to explore the local norms and values that caregivers use to justify their efforts—how Sophia talked about caring *because* Vicente was her husband—while simultaneously considering how embracing these values paradoxically gives rise to caregivers' suffering. This approach represents another dimension of the segre-social dynamics I have sought to describe throughout this book. As caregivers embrace local values to be a part of the community, their commitments risk them being misunderstood and segregated from it. Caregivers not only suffer because of the structural, social, and economic inequities that give rise to migration and related cultural change, but also because of the voices within the community that tend to blame caregivers for elders' decline. Community members understand age-related forgetfulness as a modern condition that arises because of family neglect. Hence, the local values that individuals maintain in providing care come to represent an additional cause for their suffering. I develop this argument sequentially. In the first section, I explore local values caregivers cite to justify their commitments to elders. Values concerning *familismo* and understandings about death help further account for why caregivers devote themselves to forgetful elders and the nature of responsibility that they experience. These are analyzed in terms of broader social change, and adhering to them is representative of caregivers' implicit attempts to maintain social cohesion. Yet as I show in the following section, adhering to these values in the home paradoxically risks undermining caregivers' standing in the broader community. These together represent the segre-social dynamics inherent to their experience—the way in which caregivers simultaneously form new relationships at home, and risk suffering from lack of ones in the community. In light of Sophia's loneliness, I discuss how caregiving has potential to render individuals into a second forgotten subject, now forgotten by the community whose customs they uphold. This is a central reason for why caregivers suffer and for the loneliness they endure.

LOCAL VALUES AND CAREGIVING RESPONSIBILITY: "IF THAT HAPPENS, OUR PROBLEMS WILL NEVER END"

Sophia reflected on the importance of family cohesion and how pursing this value came at the expense of her personal happiness. During the time he was healthy, Sophia felt oppressed and frightened by Vicente's abuse. But she did not want to jeopardize how her children viewed their father. "I felt relieved when my children left," Sophia said about when the last of her children migrated to California. "Even though it was only the two of us, it didn't matter what he did to me. Whatever he did to me, I kept it to myself. Because I felt very bad when they lived with us and they saw me suffer." Sophia did not want her children to be worried about her, and her main concern was directed toward the cohesion of her family. She sacrificed one desire for the pursuit of another, and this choice grew to be more important with the majority of her children living so far away. She reflected on what would have happened had she told her children about the abuse she endured. At that time, she said:

> I felt as if my soul was going to tear apart. Because I wouldn't feel good if they disrespected their father. And I wouldn't let it happen anyway. . . . Because elders taught us this way, and my mom used to tell me, "Don't put a stick or rock in the hands of your kids." So I learned that whatever is happening to you, don't tell them, because they could disrespect or hurt their father. And if that happens, our problems will never end. And it will only bring on more problems. That's why I never told them what was happening to me.

The cohesion of Sophia's family was at stake—and regeneratively put in a new light as they tried to maintain it across borders. Telling her children of the abuse she endured would only give them reason to challenge their father and further disrupt family life. Sophia considers what elders have taught her, to not equip new generations with reasons to betray older ones. Family disputes and social discord is a problem that does not end. So, Sophia chose to remain silent about the abuse she endured in order to avoid a situation she wanted to prevent more.

To maintain family cohesion, Sophia decided to care for Vicente and remain quiet. Valuing cohesion over her own well-being helps put into focus caregivers' reasons to devote themselves to caring for dependent elders. In his handbook on dementia caregiving, Richard Schulz (2000) discusses the importance of responsibility and identifies egoistic, altruistic, and social norms as the various reasons for why individuals feel responsible (pp. 33–38). Schultz's discussion of social norms is most relevant here, presented as a contextualizing factor for why caregivers feel accountable to provide care. Social norms are shared expectations and standards for relationships, and Schulz rightly observes that these differ across time and space. In Oaxaca, where the household is regarded as the primary social unit, one's sense of responsibility is so often directed to this end.

Here social norms are based around shared values like familismo and *colectivismo*, crystalizing one's sense of obligation, loyalty, and sacrifice for the good of the larger social unit (Behnke et al., 2008; Calzada et al., 2013; Cervantes, 2008). With regard to caregiving for dementia, familismo has been studied to show how individuals make decisions about institutionalization (Gaugler, Kane, Kane, & Newcomer, 2006), how it is a factor leading to caregiver distress (Robinson Shurgot & Knight, 2005), and how it modifies family members' perceptions of available social support (Gelman, 2012).

This set of research is helpful for contextualizing Sophia's decision to care for Vicente, but it does not go far enough to account for how her reasons engage with and negotiate values in the process. In Sophia's case, her decision to assume responsibility for Vicente involved wanting to maintain family cohesion in the context of when it seemed most at stake. This changes what it means to assume responsibility for elders and why these reasons are felt with such importance. Indeed, how values change and the way these changes impact reasons to be responsible is implicit even in the language caregivers use to describe responsibility itself. Although there exist other words to refer to "responsibility," *responsabl*, a Spanish cognate, is the Zapotec word Sophia and other caregivers used most frequently.[1] Adopting a Spanish word in everyday Zapotec is but one linguistic illustration of the much more diffuse ways that language and values in Teotitlán continue to evolve and engage with other cultural influences, and how this larger social evolution redefines the meaning of caring for dependent elders. Caregivers accept responsibility not only for the purposes of sustaining the lives of loved ones, but also for the ways that this dedication affirms key values many believe are endangered today.

One common way that caregivers justified their responsibility was through appealing to local notions about familismo and elders' place in the family. In Sophia's case, she described how she cared for Vicente *because* it was expected of her role as a wife. Yet given the difficulties she endured, I asked Sophia about why she did not find a way to ask other family members or friends for help. "Because he wouldn't want it," she said, "and I wouldn't let that happen." Once again, it seemed almost a given that their relationship justified Sophia's assumption of responsibility.

Indeed, other caregivers cited similar rationales and helped further explain how assuming responsibility for elders was part and parcel of what it meant to be related. This duty, this responsibility inherent to relatedness, is a fact Mario also considered as he cared for his father, Nicholas (discussed in chapter 3).

Recovering from a stroke, Nicholas was now incontinent and largely dependent on family care. Curious about how he justified his effort and time, I asked about how Mario understood his responsibility. Here, Isabelle responds on behalf of Mario, her husband (who at this time found this topic emotionally difficult). She said, "What he tells me is that 'We will all get to be old. And my dad is getting old that way. So I have to take care of him. I have to take care of him to the best of my ability.' He accepts the situation." Isabelle's summarizing statement that Mario "accepts the situation" does not just refer to accepting his father's condition, but is also expressive of his view of the aging process itself. It is recognition that all people grow old if they live long enough. And that Mario might experience a condition similar to his father's—old, unable to work, and in need of care. Just like Mario would want to be cared for in his future dependency, he identifies and feels responsible for his father who experiences it now.[2] He expresses a hope, a vision of the future where there will be someone like him to assume responsibility for himself in old age. But in a climate marked by social fragmentation, Mario implicitly knows it is something he cannot count on. How Mario values familismo is constituted by experience in a world that increasingly seems to undermine it.

To further understand this perspective I wondered about nursing homes and why caregivers do not consider professional care as an option. There are three nursing homes for elders, two government-funded homes and a privately funded one. They are subsidized but still questionably affordable.[3] Though these homes bar persons with dementia by requiring that new residents have the cognitive capacity to be aware that they are relocating, during my visits to these homes I encountered multiple cases of elders who later grew to develop symptoms. These facilities are not oriented toward treating dementia, but it seemed possible that forgetful elders could be cared for here.

Local perspectives of sending elders to nursing homes was discussed among Carlos and Francisco, when I made a comment that the intensity of their experience caring for Cynthia with late-stage Alzheimer's might have been alleviated through professional help. The family explained why such options were infeasible.

> CARLOS: Well, to begin, in Oaxaca nursing homes are very new. Secondly, the custom that we guide ourselves by [is that] until the person has passed away, that's when you are no longer relatives. For instance, she's my wife. So until she dies that's when she is no longer my wife. That's a custom. It is shameful if you take your relative to a nursing

home. And also [your] conscience would not be at peace. At least on my part, I would not be in peace if I were to take her there. Because I don't know how she would be treated. Even though she's like that, she is cared for here—by all of us.

FRANCISCO: No I wouldn't be able to do it either. And also like [my father] said, because of our customs, that's just not possible. And it's not viewed well by the community, if you were to take an elder to a nursing home.

CARLOS: And also your conscience wouldn't be at peace.

FRANCISCO: And also because we've spent so much time with her, it would be difficult to do it.

Carlos observes what every other caregiver implicitly knows—that nursing homes are new and that viewing care as a commodity is not part of local thinking. Professional caregiving contrasts with local notions about what it means to have an elder in one's family. It means that you have someone to take care of. This is illustrated in Carlos's statement about his wife being a family member until her death, and how this fact entails his responsibility for her. Hence, the very definition of family—and the way in which Carlos continues to view his wife as a part of his family—presupposes an obligation to care. This is what brings his family together. "Even though she's like that, she is cared for here—by all of us," he says. Care itself is representative of the cohesion he wants.[4]

Yet while all these ideas involve caregivers' relationships with elders at home, they also coalesce around broader concerns with the community. Carlos and Francisco imagine that a failure to care for Cynthia would be perceived by others as a larger failure of upholding shared values about how to treat elders. They imagine being judged, shamed, and having a conscience "not at peace." In this way, beyond compromising family cohesion, seeking professional help would also lead to a broader loss in standing within the community. Maintaining cohesion in the home is also a way to engage with the community outside. It is a public statement about one's commitment to the family and, by extension, one's commitment to common values. This provides more context to Sophia's determination to care for Vicente; among her family in California who might otherwise lose their ties to Teotitlán, upholding these values is constitutive of what it means to belong to the broader community. So too, with Carlos and Francisco. "It's just not possible," Francisco says, to imagine being a Teotiteco and acting otherwise. The problems that "will never end" are social ones, ramifications of not pursuing this collective good.

Caregivers also cited other reasons to justify their responsibility that do not involve familismo, but ideas about death and dying. Similar to the perspectives featured above, this invokes concerns about social cohesion at a time when it seems most at stake. For example, Carlos's twice-repeated statement of having a bad conscience was about the idea of admitting his wife to a nursing home, but it also hinted at local ideas about his relationship with Cynthia once she passed. Carlos does not want to regret overlooking his responsibility as a husband, a feeling that he believes would haunt him throughout his subsequent life. Similarly, Sophia hinted at this perspective when she quoted her brother who implored her to not have regrets with Vicente, and to care for him to the best of her ability. "I will not regret anything," she said with determination.

In previous pages I began to discuss how, instead of marking the end of relationships, in Oaxaca death is known to initiate a new type of relationship, leading to a new set of social responsibilities, commitments, and interpersonal connections that extend beyond the lifetime of the deceased. With the exception of children (angelitos, literally "angels") who ascend directly to heaven—and severe sinners who go directly to hell—the majority of deceased adults are thought to have souls that exist in a liminal purgatory state, needing to undergo a period of penitence in order to be purified to gain access to heaven.[5] Living people are expected to carry out regular actions on behalf of the deceased to help toward this end, praying for them to gain salvation and demonstrating to the deceased that they have not been forgotten. If successful, their souls are said to return to the community on the Day of the Dead, a celebration to mark when the deceased have completed their journeys through purgatory and gained access to heaven. In Teotitlán, like the majority of settings in Oaxaca, some of these customs are practiced on a daily level, both during the purgatory period and well after the soul is believed to have arrived in heaven. Most homes have an altar for paying respect to deceased persons—with photographs of deceased family members, accompanied by flowers, candles, and other offerings—and individuals are expected to pay homage here and regularly visit family gravesites. As Kristen Norget (2006) beautifully describes in her study of Oaxacan death customs, remembering the deceased brings family and the larger community together, creating a sense of belonging through unified work on behalf of the dead. This regenerates cohesion, and gives the deceased power in maintaining cohesion in the family. In this way, writes Norget, "life and death are not viewed as mutually exclusive ontological states. Death is not experienced as an event that introduces discontinuity and disruption. . . . [Rather,] the dead are understood

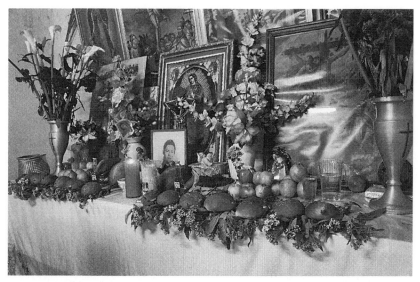

FIG. 5.1. Home altar with offerings during Day of the Dead. *Photograph by Michelle Nermon. Used with permission.*

to return frequently to the domain of the living" (pp. 115–16; see also Royce, 2011). Through their presence in the community, the dead help revitalize and maintain social cohesion.

This perspective is representative of an additional reason caregivers feel responsible to care for forgetful elders. This was most clearly articulated by Francisca and her daughter, Dominga, the caregivers introduced in the previous chapter who described the alarming experience of witnessing Antonio's seizures and other memory losses associated with his stoke history. At one point, Francisca recalled a recent exchange she had with Antonio and how she spoke to him as if he were already dead. Francisca's summary provides greater perspective of how local understandings about death justify her responsibility to care for Antonio now.

> And like I told [Antonio], for instance yesterday when I was talking to him. [*Francisca begins to whisper.*] "I believe that you realize now that you're not with us anymore. I don't know what you feel, or where you are, or where you feel you are. Or, I don't know what you feel about where you are"—since he always says that when he dreams he is on a path, and that he is leaving, or going away—"So I ask you

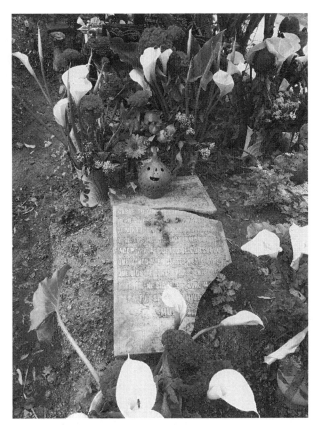

FIG. 5.2. Gravesite during Day of the Dead. *Photograph by the author.*

for just one little thing, Antonio, if you pass away in this condition," I told him, "it will not be our fault. And you know that we have taken care of you the best we can. I did not despise you," I told him. "I never left you alone in any festivity or party, I never left you hungry. . . . At the moment that you receive God's will [Zapotec original: *dixtxey* "God's gift of death," but also a "gift" in general], go freely and peacefully. I don't want you to return and bother us. Because there are people that, when they die in this way, return and bother their relatives. I assume you have lived a good life, so please forget everything you've been through, or anything that's happened to you." That's what I told him.

Francisca's words help illustrate how anticipation of Antonio's death in the future leads to feelings of responsibility for him in the present. She views Antonio in the process of dying, speaks to him as half-dead, and begs him to leave the family in peace. Though the dead have been known for returning peacefully to the community of the living, Francisca illustrates how they also might come to haunt and burden it. This occurs when deceased people were not treated well by family or did not die peacefully. So, Francisca tries to mitigate this risk, to remind Antonio that he has had a good life and that she and Dominga have done everything in their power to provide for him during his illness. In part, she cares for Antonio now to serve her family later.

This helps further explain Sophia's perspective and her brother's suggestion that she cares for Vicente to the best of her ability. The importance of providing a good death and properly caring for the dying represent an additional reason for how and why caregivers experience responsibility as a matter of serving the larger family. Whereas caregivers uphold notions of familismo to maintain a sense of cohesion with elders now, their anticipation of elders' death is an equal concern for the family unit later. "Death does not threaten social order, so much as provide an occasion to revitalize it," writes Norget (2006, p. 114). It encourages living persons to exist in harmony and to behave in a manner that honors the deceased. The caregivers I studied confirm and deepen this observation by showing how even the anticipation of death revitalizes moral behavior and the importance of family cohesion. "If not a good life, then a 'good death,' " writes Norget (p. 115); and, caregivers implicitly add, "if not a good death marked by an elder's wisdom and authority, then good care and good family while anticipating it." Together, these notions about how one ought to die and the importance of properly caring for elders shape the meaning and rationale of caregiving. They illustrate how caregiving responsibility is constituted by and oriented toward a larger notion of the good that is centered on family and social cohesion. Caregivers organize their lives and structure their family toward the pursuit of this good, simultaneously illustrating how social relations in the home are organized by social values outside, and how those values exist in light of broader changes to the community.

THE SECOND FORGOTTEN SUBJECT: "PERHAPS IT'S NOT TRUE THAT HE IS ILL"

"I need to talk so I can relax my mind," Sophia said. "[But] no one has come and asked me how I'm doing, like 'How are you doing taking care of him?' Someone who could empathize with me, or someone who could just give me a word of

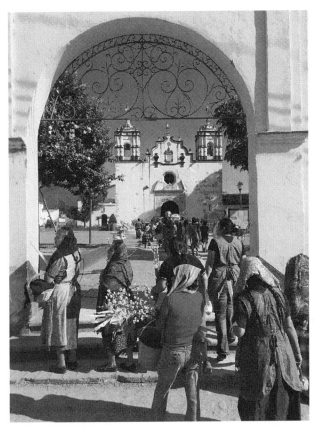

FIG. 5.3. Funeral procession. *Photograph by the author.*

hope. That's something that would comfort me." Indeed, the comfort Sophia sought was juxtaposed to the loneliness she felt. Though her children were aware of Vicente's condition—and though Sophia saw other family and friends in the community—she felt alone. She explained how people did not understand her experience as caregiver and, further, she sensed that she was misunderstood for it. This may come as a surprise given how Sophia and other caregivers justified their responsibility through appealing to values of the community. As other researchers have described the paradoxes that arise in caregivers' attempts to maintain local values in the context of transnational migration—for example, Parreñas's (2005) description of a "gender paradox" that arises in transnational circumstances where gender norms are simultaneously redefined and reinforced—Sophia highlighted the way in which striving for family cohesion can paradoxically render caregivers on the social periphery.

This paradox is perhaps best articulated through attending to the segre-social dynamics that caregivers experience. Caregivers are drawn into new social forms by caring for forgetful elders, first, in how caregivers themselves rearrange social arrangements at home and come together to provide care and, second, by how caregivers relate to elders. As discussed in the previous chapter, the latter represents a significant shift from how elders are traditionally viewed via their authority and life wisdom, toward how caregivers come to relate to elders' via their dependencies and need for care. This relational shift challenges the local meaning of aging, but it simultaneously affirms local values about family and social cohesion. Caregivers would be stigmatized if they did not uphold these values and provide necessary care for elders. And yet, in a setting where age-related forgetfulness is indexed to broader notions of social change—where Alzheimer's is believed to not exist and forgetfulness is caused by modern stress—caregivers risk being held accountable for elders' decline. While caregiving represents a new form of social life, caregivers simultaneously face social isolation when it comes to the rest of the community's perception of them. The paradox is that while caregivers avoid stigma by embracing local values through caring for elders, caregivers risk encountering another stigma in being blamed for the condition they are trying to treat.

To begin developing this point I pause and return to consider how Sophia's loneliness contrasts with common notions of Teotiteco citizenship, and how local belonging is typically associated with social support. As I have discussed throughout this book, this is the case not just in Teotitlán, but throughout Oaxaca where the household—not the individual—is the primary social unit; people regularly understand themselves through the family and broader socio-familial frameworks (J. Cohen, 2004; Murphy & Stepick, 1991; Norget, 2006). This is why Sophia's loneliness is so important to attend to.

Yet Sophia was not the only caregiver to experience loneliness, and I encountered the majority of other households with similar sentiments. Mario, Isabelle, and Graciela described feeling forgotten by the rest of their family because these members did not live with them and failed to show appreciation for their daily caregiving experience. Mario, for example, has brothers in California and Teotitlán, "but they only come every now and then. And there are days that they don't come at all," he says. "It's very seldom when they come." Like Sophia, their experience of being confined at home carries an additional dimension of loneliness: unable to leave home and socialize in the community, Mario described also feeling forgotten by extended members of his family.

This also includes caregivers' relationships with fictive kinship networks established through the *compadrazgo* system. As mentioned prior, Sergio, Manuel, and Linda described their positive relationships with godchildren and how they saw them on important holidays, but similarly described feeling alone in the everyday experience of caregiving. "Each person has their own way of doing things," Manuel said while talking about his godchildren, "and so they can't be obligated to come." These statements may appear marginal, but they importantly shape the everyday experience of caregiving and the loneliness associated with it.

While caregivers experience loneliness in the context of immediate and extended families, they also spoke of isolation in the larger community owing to being the topic of local gossip. Like in most rural communities, news travels quickly in Teotitlán, and members are prone to talking about one another. Gossip is a daily occurrence in Teotitlán, and I witnessed people gossiping about a myriad of topics—including my presence in the community—throughout fieldwork. Gossip, I came to realize, seemed to be part and parcel of social life. For example, the public market is locally known not only as a site to purchase household goods, but also for being a place to socialize through gossip. It is *puro chisme* (Spanish: pure gossip), people repeatedly told me through laughter. The Zapotec phrase for speaking gossip—*nalu dambur*—further sheds light on its nature, a phrase that refers to a person who parades through the streets while clanging on a tambourine to announce community events. In Teotitlán, gossip is not something one can easily ignore, but rather a significant way people are held accountable to—and participate within—the community.[6]

Initially, anthropologists understood gossip as a mechanism of social control; in being subject (or subjecting another) to it, gossip facilitates social cohesion by holding people accountable to surrounding social rules (Gluckman, 1963). Yet as John Haviland (1977) quickly observed in his research in Mexico, gossip does not merely enforce social rules, but *creates* them. "If we observe gossips in action we soon understand that one does not just appeal to norms or rules; rather, one applies them, manipulates them, and interprets them for particular purposes. Gossiping requires such manipulation of rules" (p. 17). In this way, gossip is a practice that regenerates social norms, highlighting relevant social rules in a given circumstance, and demonstrates their continued value through holding others accountable to them.

Caregivers' concern about gossip was one reason why conducting this ethnography was challenging. Most individuals lacked *confianza* (confidence or trust) that they could speak to Alex (a member of the community who might create further gossip) or me (a foreigner to the community who might misunderstand them). In one instance, Carlos and his family debated inviting us into their home for months. Though this was the most extreme challenge gaining access, all caregivers showed some degree of concern speaking to us. This was something Pablo explicitly talked about, comparing his decision to invite us to his home to the restraint he imagined most other caregivers showed us. "I've often traveled so I got to know other people," he said distinguishing himself from others. "I'm more open-minded and I'm able to share my thoughts. Because if you were to go to someone else's house, they would rather close their doors. Or they would just say that they don't want to be interviewed." The private experience of caregiving was not something people readily wanted to discuss publicly.

Others provided more insight about why caregivers wanted to remain quiet about their experience. They discussed how they sensed they were the topic of gossip, and how such talk implicitly blamed them for elders' decline. For example, Francisca and Dominga talked about the lack of understanding they experience in the broader community and how it contributed to their isolation. In doing their best to manage Antonio's confusion and behavioral outbursts, they decided to limit how much he went out in public. But this caused others to gossip about them. At one point, Francisca said:

> And now, what happens to him, which wouldn't have happened before [his illness]. . . . If he were to go out, he'd get scared. . . . He'd scream. . . . He'd run. And that happened [before] so many times. [So] we locked him up. But, God forgive me, you know how our relatives are. So they say, "Perhaps it's not true that he is ill."

People contrasted how they knew Antonio as a respected elder in the community to the character they last saw—disoriented, frightened, and forgetful. To manage their impressions and keep Antonio safe, they decided to minimize these public scenes. But in the process, neighbors and family members have begun to notice his absence and question whether he is actually ill or if, they gossiped, Francisca and Dominga are actually to blame. "There are people that say we don't care about what's going on with my uncle. But that's a lie," Dominga added. "They don't really know what's inside of you. They will never know what someone's intentions really are."

Similar to this experience, Sergio, Manuel, and Linda also discussed concerns about being the topic of gossip. As they spoke among themselves about their "tricky" father, they illustrated how they regularly try to manage people's impressions, and how gossip has come to be a central concern regarding the way they socialize in the community.

> SERGIO: When people see him walking out [on the street], they probably
> think we don't properly take care of him.
> MANUEL: Sometimes people criticize elders, or their relatives that [don't]
> take care of them. For instance, him, when he goes out—and since
> he doesn't like to shower—people might say that we don't take care
> of him properly.
> SERGIO: I've even talked to people his age, and I talk to them and tell them
> about him. . . . And in the end they often tell us that we're the ones
> that are not taking care of him properly.
> MANUEL: The way people view elders is determined by how they think
> their children are taking care of them.
> LINDA: I tell him to change his clothes.
> MANUEL: And a lot of people criticize us, the way we take care of him.
> Because that's the way it seems from the outside. We're the ones that do
> not take care of him the way we're supposed to. And that's the way people
> in town are. They don't know what's really going on. And everything
> that's happening inside they can't see. And sometimes we [the commu-
> nity] tend to criticize, and we don't understand how things really are.

As Manuel observes through his own experience caring for his father, an elder's disheveled appearance can mean two different things, depending on one's perspective. For caregivers like him, it is representative of the ongoing challenges they encounter and how their relationships with elders have evolved. Yet for the larger community it is suggestive of family mistreatment. Manuel's succinct statement—"everything that's happening inside they can't see"—at once testifies to the experience he knows others are blind to, and the way in which this dual reality creates misunderstanding among his neighbors. This misunderstanding is constitutive of Manuel's isolation, and how he and other caregivers can be blamed by the community for a condition they are trying their best to care for.[7] In upholding their commitment to care for his father, Manuel and his family are reinforcing communal values about social cohesion and respect for elders. But in the process, the gossip they are subject to regenerates the meaning of those values. Gossip seems to reemphasize the importance of social cohesion in a setting where people are liable to jettison it. In Manuel's words, "the way people view elders is determined by how they think their children are taking care of them." This is a contrast to how elders are perceived simply on account of their accumulated life experience and wisdom.

Of course, people gossip because they are concerned for elders—that elders remain respected and treated as such—and that families are upholding their responsibilities. But in so doing, gossip creates a division among the community. As people unify through gossip to agree that elders ought to be well treated and families ought to be cohesive, gossip also seems to imply that caregivers might not uphold these values. In this way, the community becomes defined through a standard that some citizens uphold, but others might disregard. This complicates classical depictions of how group cohesion is maintained in the presence of illness. Typically, representations of illness are understood as a mechanism groups use to affirm their identity. People living with illness are seen as different from the rest of a social group, and this perceived difference reinforces a sense of cohesion among the rest of the community (see Jodelet, 1991). Yet in Teotitlán, the one who is different is not the disheveled and ill person (not the forgetful elder); rather it is the caregiver who is considered responsible for causing the elder's forgetfulness. Caregivers are viewed as the exception to the social group, cast aside because of their perceived negligence of communal values. In the process, the community comes together through reaffirming the importance of cohesion and respect for elders, but does so through identifying caregivers as the individuals who do not live by these standards.

Implicit in Sophia's loneliness was awareness of how others perceived her. Indeed, while she talked about caregiving as a type of sacrifice made on behalf of her husband, Sophia and other caregivers also spoke of it as an instance of suffering. Sophia's sacrifice involved giving herself to caring for Vicente *for the purpose* of maintaining family cohesion and her commitment to him. People can make sense of sacrifices like this; they have a purpose and function. But the suffering she spoke of is distinct because it has no purpose. Sophia's experience of loneliness is not framed as serving a purpose, but something she simply endures. It is suffering in its etymological sense—illustrating the meaning of the old French verb *sofrir*, pointing to a situation one bears and endures. Suffering is thus teleologically distinct from sacrifice; whereas sacrifice involves enduring something for the purpose of a specific end, suffering has no such justification. Philosopher Emmanuel Levinas (1998a) famously writes that suffering is "useless" because it is "for nothing." It is something one senselessly endures and, because of this nature, it is unsettling to witness another person experience. Levinas goes on to develop an ethics based on this encounter—when a person witnesses another suffering, that person faces the experience of being singularly accountable to respond.[8] This is yet another dimension of why suffering is social in nature: witnessing it invokes a responsibility to do something about it; suffering fosters a social response. And, this is why recent writings in anthropology have described caregiving and suffering as being made of the same experiential fabric: "like social suffering, caregiving makes unavoidable the interrelationship between subjectivity and society," write Wilkinson and Kleinman (2016). "Both point to the interpersonal space as the context where human life and life projects succeed and fail, where human beings endure" (p. 162).

This is not just a theoretical detour, but one that more importantly helps explain the broader nature of this book. Through meeting different caregivers and learning of their isolation, I began to realize that conducting research was, at key moments, a positive experience for caregivers that occasioned the social contact they lacked. It was a way to respond to their suffering. This is perhaps best illustrated through Alex's response to Sophia when he went beyond his role as a research assistant and conveyed his understanding as a member of their shared community. The most telling instance occurred when Sophia began to cry while talking about her fear of being alone and widowed.

ALEX: Don't feel bad that you're crying—it's good that you're crying. That's one of the reasons that we're here. It helps people to cry.

JON: Tell her that I know it's really difficult, and I really appreciate that she's able to talk to us about it.

ALEX: He is thanking you that you're giving us the privilege to interview you. And like I said, this is a good way to help people get out their feelings. Because sometimes we close ourselves up, or there are people—like our own relatives—who don't understand us. If you are sharing [your feelings] with someone, they [might not] listen to you. They will always have something [else] to say. [But] we won't say anything to you. All we are saying is listening. And it will help because you're getting out everything you have inside.

Alex goes beyond translating my words to compose his own. He responds as a member of Sophia's community, acknowledging the isolation he now knows her to experience and providing her the comfort he knows is relevant. He gives her the occasion to be heard. He invites her to cry. And, in so doing, he expresses his understanding of the project and its purpose in the community, embodying what many researchers have sought in calling for a more activist style of inquiry: he does research to make a difference.[9]

This response also conveys a certain type of empathy. Yet in contrast to how empathy is commonly taken to suggest a shared horizon of meaning between two people, Alex's empathy cannot be understood without attending to its more complicated nature, what anthropologists have described as the "broader context of the ways in which people gain knowledge of others and reveal, allow, or conceal knowledge of themselves" (Hollan & Throop, 2008, p. 389). Alex's response to Sophia is thus mediated not just by the fact that he observes her suffering, but that Sophia chooses to disclose particular aspects of her suffering—and that Alex positions himself as being attentive to listen. As Alex realizes the ways cohesion in his community has been fragmented among caregivers, his response reinvokes and regenerates his value of it. As he sees it, we have been visiting caregivers to alleviate their emotional pain, to facilitate self-expression, and to feel understood within the community. Our approach is to simply listen, to not talk back, to not criticize, and cease minimizing caregivers' experience. Conducting this research is to give Sophia and other caregivers what Alex has realized they lack—a sense of being cared for themselves. In Alex's own words, "All we are saying is listening."

In part, Alex's response is expressive of the broader social changes occurring within his community. As Whitney Duncan (2018) observes, in Oaxaca the idea that expressing emotions is a positive way to manage distress is an instance of what she terms "psychological modernization," the popularization of Euro-American ideas about mental health that stand in juxtaposition to local ones. Whereas in Oaxaca, expression of one's emotions was formerly thought to be illness-producing (Hunt, 1992, p. 310; Norget, 2006, p. 86), Alex's response is indicative of a shift where self-expression is now viewed as a means toward its alleviation. Yet valuing self-expression also gains traction in places like Teotitlán because it helps make sense of—and respond to—changes within the community. Given my background in psychology, I could not help but reflect on how self-expression is also a way for caregivers to be understood in a setting where they felt so isolated. Talk is so central to the treatment I am trained to provide, as it is to the way people forge connections in broader arenas of everyday life. In this way, while Alex's words are expressive of modernizing projects, I cannot also consider how they are also representative of a socially engaged response to the circumstances he has come to recognize within his own community.

The resonance of Alex's statement can be measured by Sophia's reaction to it. Empathy not only involves Alex's experience of understanding Sophia, but her experience of feeling understood by him (see Hollan, 2008). Though I initially considered ending our discussion because it appeared to cause Sophia distress, my clinical training led me to intuit that Sophia's crying was not a request to stop talking, but an expression of gratitude to be invited to it. Intense emotion like what I encountered with Sophia can be sensitively held, and sometimes offering a space for its expression is the most appropriate response one can give. Drawing on this sensibility, I came to realize that this discussion gave Sophia an opportunity to describe her experience in a way she had not before, an occasion to be heard in the context of a community at times deaf to it. To this point, Sophia later came to say:

> Those questions [you] asked helped me to get everything out. It's just like when you're talking to someone and getting everything you have inside out. After that, you're more relaxed. And [through doing it] I feel stronger. That's the way I experienced it. That's the way I experienced it, because I need someone to talk to. I need to talk so I can relax my mind. . . . Thank you for everything, and all the questions you asked. You have left me happy. . . . After all, I think God sent you. I don't know how, but there's a reason why you came. Things don't happen—there's always a reason why things happen. God always sends someone to give hope and strength. . . . It's my hope for me to get through this hard time, and to relieve my soul. And right now the questions you asked, I gladly answered them. For instance, when I go somewhere, I like to talk, and I like to share my thoughts. And I believe that doing so relieves my mind and helps me be happy. I don't like being sad. Because if I get depressed, or if something happens to me, I will probably die before him [*Sophia laughs*]. That's why I thank you.

Sophia made clear that these sentiments were not just directed toward me and my initiating this encounter, but also toward Alex as a representative of the community. She repeatedly used the plural form of the word "you" as, for example, when she said *xtiusenyubtuu*, the Zapotec phrase for "thank you" addressed in the plural (and never *xtiuseniubiu*, the phrase in the singular). Alex bearing witness to Sophia's experience is the relevant response to learning her story. It brings these two individuals together in a moment when Alex realizes they have been rendered apart. In this way, Sophia's gratitude is only understandable in context to the larger isolation she faces. Distinct from her sense of sacrifice for her husband, Sophia's loneliness was a suffering that did not serve a larger purpose. The interview was a response to that realization, and provided an exception to the isolation she faces on a daily basis. Indeed, the gratitude Sophia expressed was not unique, and the majority of my meetings with caregivers culminated in invitations to return to their homes, and unplanned affectionate encounters in public settings. Though Sophia was the only caregiver who alone held responsibility for a dependent elder, she put into focus a loneliness—a suffering—that was palpable throughout my fieldwork, both inside the homes I studied and outside the ones that were too guarded to speak.

~

The paradox in these observations is that while caregiving can be understood as a practice that embraces values concerning social cohesion, locals' perception of caregivers also might entail their social isolation. In this chapter I have explored the values that sustain caregiving practice—values concerning familismo, death, and dying—and how they help foster greater social cohesion and serve to engage with the broader community. I have also discussed how the community is liable to blame caregivers for elders' forgetfulness and related behavioral decline that they interpret to be caused by modern stress and related social change, conditions that ultimately are seen as the family's responsibility to prevent. In the process, I have shown how caregivers can become rendered into a second forgotten subject, forgotten and misunderstood by a community whose values they do their best to embrace. This is illustrative of the segre-social dynamics of local caregiving experience. Caregiving at once represents novel social forms, both as caregivers relate to forgetful elders in new ways and come together themselves as they strategize to distribute responsibilities at home. Were it not for these efforts, families would be stigmatized for failing to respect and care for elders. Yet caregiving also might lead to segregation. Age-related forgetfulness is indexed to broader social change, where failures concerning the latter are understood as a cause for the former. This is the social suffering that caregivers endure, where their "embodied experience is held up as a mirror to [a] society" that is negotiating the meaning of—and response to—social change (Wilkinson & Kleinman, 2016, p. 14). Attending to the lived experience of caregiving puts these social dynamics in focus.

Epilogue

Every year, after the somber processions of Easter but before the torrential rains of summer, the people of Teotitlán assemble for a five-day fiesta. Brass bands parade through the streets, costumed dancers cavort in the public plaza, and different households across the community unite. Although popularly referred to as *carnival*, this event is also known for a more specific name, *La Danza de los Viejos* (The Dance of the Elders).[1]

In fact, in this *Danza* actual elders of the community are not the main participants, but rather a group of youths in costume meant to represent old age. With grayed whiskers and sunken eyes, each afternoon two young men don wooden masks to conceal their identities. These *viejitos* (affectionate elders) begin slowly, theatrically limping over wooden canes and lumbering through the streets.[2] The elders' wives—also men in costume—shriek in laughter as a throng of people, with a brass band following, head toward the municipal building.

These viejitos represent ancestors who have returned to the community to offer advice. They possess common knowledge that is otherwise unspoken; they know what has occurred behind private doors. The viejitos and their wives first meet privately with the municipal president in his office. In Teotitlán, a setting where respect is paramount—where one does not criticize authorities—what

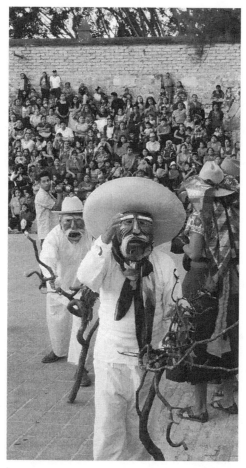

FIG. E.1. *La Danza de los Viejos. Photograph by the author.*

occurs is exceptional. In private and later in public, the viejitos identify shortcom-
ings, embezzlements, and even illicit affairs. They tell the president what he has
done wrong and what the community is lacking. And, after each critique, gossip,
or joke, the viejitos' wives erupt in cackled laughter that echoes throughout the
streets. Anyone is target to their gossip and, during the community dance that
follows, the elders slowly turn their attention to the broader group of spectators.[3]
Their ribald jokes and quick criticisms are contagious. Their caricature of old
age is uproarious.

And yet, for all its levity and despite all the fun, this rendition provides a more profound image of what old age means in Teotitlán today. It is an image where elders' authority is matched with farce, where the *bengul* who is seen as a bastion of tradition now becomes a spectacle of entertainment. Of course, locals know that this is a staged affair. But the fact that this provides such occasion for laughter—that the viejitos can so captivatingly foment such fun—demonstrates that the traditional black-and-white picture of the bengul is better represented in shades of gray. This is the spectrum through which some elders are seen in Teotitlán, the ambivalence experienced by a community that views itself at once anchored by idealized notions of tradition and threatened to be adrift by a simultaneous engagement with modernity.

The anthropologist Michael Jackson (2017) writes that the "work of rituals" promotes an expression of ambivalence in a form that simultaneously affirms solidarity and like-mindedness (p. 9). This book has put into focus underlying ambivalence about contemporary life and subsequent responses to it, revealing how caregivers attempt to uphold local identity and values—all while situated in a broader social world where identity continually evolves and values are regenerated. I suspect all communities evolve in parallel to broader world dynamics. For its part, Teotitlán is situated at its own symbolic intersection between idealized notions of tradition and modernity, where nostalgic depictions of the former are embraced through representations of social change indexed to the latter. These representations are not meant to suggest that Teotitlán is somehow experiencing a cultural shift from one period of time to another—Teotitlán is not somehow becoming any less "Teotiteco." Rather, these representations are opposite poles of the same contemporary experience, markers to make sense of the dynamics of contemporary social life. Tradition becomes important when one can envision not living traditionally. Analogously, embracing modernity only makes sense in the context of alternatives to the prioritization of capital gain and social independence—alternatives, for example, that embrace shared economies and social cohesion. The people studied in this book with their histories, encounters with different political and medical systems, and transborder family genealogies are situated in the middle of this junction: they continually negotiate how to live meaningful and dignified lives in the context of the dynamics that make up their broader social worlds.

The annual Danza is also representative of the intimate experience of caregiving itself. It represents ambivalence about how elders are cared for on the basis of their local authority, and also how that authority is questioned, negotiated, and redefined. Forgetfulness not only stands as a challenge to the way elders are normatively viewed, but also for the way it is associated with the stress of individualistic, "nontraditional" lifestyles. For most in the community, Alzheimer's (and to varying degrees, related dementias) are believed simply to not exist locally. They are modern conditions that arise in pursuit of a modern life. This was the dominant opinion held by laypersons, but also medics at the Centro de Salud, traditional healers, and political leaders. Even the majority of caregivers did not know about other households who dealt with similar instances of forgetfulness. Forgetfulness represents an undermining of sociofamilial cohesion, a decline in elders' authority of local wisdom, and an overall transformation of broader identity. Again, this is not to suggest that life in Teotitlán is somehow shifting from one temporal category to another. Rather, the social dynamics that constitute forgetfulness and those who care for the forgetful are representative of how people form a sense of community in everyday contemporary life.

Overall, this book has highlighted how individuals come together through acts of care to affirm and regenerate the meaning of local values. The functional, pragmatic nature of caregivers' idioms of distress used to account for forgetfulness—their perceptions of what constitutes forgetfulness and their etiological understandings for why it occurs—put into focus how local perspectives about forgetfulness arise in pursuit of values perceived to be endangered by it. Caregivers' perception and speculation about underlying causes of forgetfulness help reintegrate elders and maintain family cohesion. In this way, the meaning of forgetfulness is not only constructed within current social circumstances, but also constructive of the world in which caregivers aspire to live. Similarly, in attending to health-seeking behaviors, caregivers demonstrate how their decisions to consult medical providers are situated in a broader sociopolitical context. While caregivers are primarily concerned with meeting elders' immediate needs, the decision to consult providers from varying medical traditions is also expressive of caregivers' broader negotiation of social factors inherent to contemporary life. This is also true of caregiving relationships. Between caregivers and forgetful elders, social relations illustrate the ambivalence inherent in providing care to dependent elders, and how these dynamics reconstitute social relations at home. Forgetful elders are simultaneously viewed as socially important persons with experience, but also dependents resembling children in need of care. Similarly, between caregivers and the larger community, as caregivers attempt to engage with the community by upholding values through providing care, they can be paradoxically overlooked because of their commitment to this goal. This is the social suffering caregivers described as they did their best to navigate between a public setting that tends to misunderstand them and a home environment that demands their attention.

The segre-social dynamics of this book are meant to account for this larger instance of how local values are constituted, regenerated, and maintained for purposes of social cohesion. The term points to how caregivers are drawn into new social relations centered on treating dementia, both in their personal relations with forgetful elders and also among themselves as they alter social arrangements at home to provide care. But, in a setting where age-related forgetfulness is indexed to broader notions of social change, caregivers can be simultaneously held accountable for elders' decline. Caregiving thus represents a new form of sociality at home, and potential for a concomitant loss of relations—a segregation—outside. The ambivalence expressed in Teotitlán's Danza—between depictions of old age as authority and farce—is mirrored by the experiences of its caregivers.

PRAGMATIC CONSIDERATIONS FOR CLINICAL PROVIDERS AND GENERAL READERS

As a clinical psychologist, I approached this book to understand the nature of culture and the social construction of aging. I viewed these two phenomena to be interrelated clinical issues. Moreover, I intuited that conducting an ethnography and engaging with anthropology would help me sensitize to the fluid ways that culture and aging are defined and experienced. And, I thought that interdisciplinary and cross-cultural research would put in perspective some of the taken-for-granted assumptions that implicitly informed my approach as a clinician and my general stance as a citizen. To be sure, this project has been instructive—in general, teaching that attending to the concrete, lived experience of culture in people's everyday lives helps foster dialogue that is genuine and knowledge that is sensitive. Such attention provides people like myself—clinicians, social researchers, and the general public—with the ability to appropriately listen and pragmatically respond. And this, I learned, is a matter not only of appreciating other people's experience, but also one's own.

Studying dementia reveals the values that are prioritized in life and the subsequent ways people choose to live. This recalls the true yet often overlooked observation that the ethnopsychiatrists taught—that any attempt to treat "abnormal" conditions is premised on a specific cultural outlook about what is believed to be normal (see Gaines, 1992). Today, in the context of pushes for detection of illness prior to manifestation of symptoms—through biomarkers and genetic analyses—this lesson seems most relevant. There is an increasing tendency to overlook the fact that the objects under the microscope are interpreted by an eye steeped in a specific cultural outlook. We ought to consider how such emphasis on neuroscience might overlook the implicit values that shape what that science comes to discover.

The experience of dementia could be different. For readers in the United States and related settings, it is significant to encounter individuals like the ones presented in this book who do not experience dementia with the same type of dread and alarm. Yes, dementia in Oaxaca signifies a certain sense of loss, but this perspective also serves to highlight communal values that foster social cohesion. This is not necessarily the case elsewhere. Indeed, as historian Jesse Ballenger (2006) writes of U.S. culture, "Dementia can be seen as one of the emblematic diseases of our times, just as hysteria was in the Victorian era" (p. 153). And, just like hysteria is intelligible only by situating it in a cultural epoch that cautioned against expressing desire, cross-cultural studies on dementia put into focus implicit values in the United States concerning self-control, self-creation, and self-determination. Losing these traits is near synonymous with losing one's personhood, as noted in the common expression that Alzheimer's is "a death that leaves the body behind." Yet the voices in this book reveal how this equation between cognitive decline and personal death is not necessarily a given. There exist other ways to experience and respond to dementia—ways that might highlight alternatives to how cognition is so prioritized that instead center on creative expression, being in the presence of others, human touch, and the myriad other dimensions to everyday experience. Celebrating these capacities could function to bring people closer together.

Being aware of implicit values that stand behind dementia and senses of personhood also highlights the ever-growing group of people who cannot uphold these values—the people with dementia and other dependencies—and how they might become cast on the social periphery. This is why Stephen Post (2000) calls Alzheimer's disease "a moral challenge." It is a challenge not because science still appears to be limited in the development of relevant medicines for the future, but rather because these values risk excluding the ill from living with dignity in the present. And further, attending to these values also highlights how people might risk overlooking something central about life itself. In the United States, illness is so often viewed as an aberration to life, and old age the foreclosure of it. Yet as historian Thomas Cole (1992) aptly points out, there is an inherent danger to tendencies that respond to the anxieties of growing old via a "psychologically primitive strategy" of splitting images of a "good" old age of health and autonomy, apart from a "bad" old age of sickness and dependency (p. 230). Doing so overlooks how health is intimately woven to moments when it is lost, how life inherently presupposes the finality of death. The caregivers in this book remind readers of an alternative: illness and death can, in themselves, be meaningful and, far from being exceptions to life, have potential to inform and deepen its meaning.

In addition to these cross-cultural perspectives, this book also highlights certain lessons about clinical care and the nature of culture itself. I began with observations from my own discipline in psychology that culture is a social category that is fluid and dynamic, and that cultural competence is a lifelong process that involves humility and openness (APA, 2017; Tervalon & Murray-Garcia, 1998). These are honest descriptions that attend to the nuanced and complicated nature of working with people from various cultural backgrounds. But the field still faces challenges. Even with suggestions on how clinicians might be trained in ethnography (Arnault & Shimabukuro, 2012; Kleinman & Benson, 2006), or APA's (2012) development of the "Cultural Formulation Interview" that directs clinicians to acquire important information about culture, mental health still seems to face difficulty incorporating cultural difference into clinical practice (see Ramírez Stege & Yarris, 2017). These difficulties appear to be based on two grounds: first, because clinicians cannot be expected to study culture with the same focus as ethnographers and, second, because defining culture as a fluid and dynamic category seems to contradict other foundational assumptions in the field. This book has attempted to address both issues by studying cultural dimensions of caregiving in Teotitlán.

First, it is true that clinicians cannot be expected to gain information about culture with the same focus that ethnography demands. I took a detour from my field to engage with others. And yet, the sensibility gained from conducting and reading ethnography demonstrates something important about culture itself: that culture significantly constitutes life experience, and that it cannot be reified to a static category that can be mastered or predicted. Clinicians should not be expected to become ethnographers, nor do they need to be ethnographers to be culturally competent. But they can and should be encouraged to maintain an ethnographic sensibility. This is a cultural pragmatism that, in part, is cultivated through reading relevant texts, gathering information about cultural backgrounds, and related inquiry. It is important to be equipped with basic cultural information so that patients feel understood and supported. But the overall point is not to master information before meeting with patients. Rather, through studying culture as a matter of dynamic fluidity, the point is to convey a desire to learn from and about people. In this way, ethnographic inquiry embodies a stance similar to the cultural pragmatism I advocated for in this book—an invitation for others to speak and for clinicians to listen. Away from mastery, certainty, and overconfidence toward openness, curiosity, and humility. This, I believe, is the real force behind all the emphasis on cultural competence in mental health, embodying so much of what it means to care in the field today.

Second, another difficulty is that maintaining this sensibility runs against other dominant assumptions in the field. As I noted at various points in this book, part of this difficulty owes to a broader epistemological inconsistency. Clinicians simultaneously appreciate how people from different cultures might varyingly experience illness, while presuming to have knowledge that transcends that experience. We might *appreciate* how age-related forgetfulness is considered normal in Teotitlán, but we limit this sensibility when ultimately claiming to *know* that there exists underlying neuropathology to better explain symptoms. Such a stance prioritizes one reality over another. It discounts what illness means on a daily level, and discredits the varying ways people might experience it.

To be sure, neurological facts matter. Empirical science matters. But so too do the cultural dimensions that dynamically constitute human experience. We face a challenge in being able to simultaneously attend to both empirical knowledge and cultural truths, in their own rights, as constituting their own respective senses of validity (see Good, 1994; Whitley, 2007). Assuming culture is something one can master through reaching a certain degree of "competence" is an attempt to apply a type of technical expertise toward a dimension of clinical work that inherently escapes that type of skill-building (Kirmayer, 2012). Being competent working with different cultures is not a matter of checking boxes off a list. And yet, in the mental-health fields, we continue to approach matters of culture in the same way as we study evidence-based research. We conflate empirical knowledge with cultural truths. This book has attempted to take this epistemological inconsistency seriously and find a way to study culture in its own terms, without making assumptions that some forms of thinking are more accurate than others. It has attempted, for example, to view the claim that Alzheimer's does not exist in Teotitlán as having cultural validity, *despite* knowledge about underlying plaques and tangles and awareness of global prevalence rates.

Reconciling this tension is difficult, and this book's approach studying cultural pragmatism is an attempt at one resolution. Indeed, while ethnography was a method to acquire information about culture, pragmatism was a theory that helped settle the epistemological inconsistency about how I came to understand it. As used in this book, pragmatism represents an epistemological shift from assuming truth as something objective across time and place, toward appreciating how various *truths* are valid because of their usefulness. Different groups of people have different reasons to come together, and studying those reasons is the key toward appreciating why different truths matter. This is what William James (1907/2000) termed the "practical cash value" of the things one holds to be true (p. 28). Things are important not because they are true in an abstract sense, but because they make a concrete difference to everyday life. Hence, pragmatism helped me approach cultural truths in themselves, without comparing or contesting them to the truths I simultaneously held. Again, to recall a point made in the introduction, my approach to pragmatism is not meant to somehow undermine scientific truths, nor to make some general declaration that all truths are socially constructed. Rather, I turned to pragmatism to "bracket" what has become a natural assumption about illness having an underlying empirical reality.

Cultural pragmatism allowed me to acknowledge how one truth might be valid for me as a clinician, and simultaneously attend to the truths of other people as well. This is because it focuses on the function of truths, and is a reminder of how those functions differ in time and place. As philosopher Richard Rorty (1982) writes on this point:

> Our identification with our community—our society, our political tradition, our intellectual heritage—is heightened when we see this community as *ours* rather than *nature's*, *shaped* rather than *found*, one among many which men have made. In the end, the pragmatists tell us, what matters is our loyalty to other human beings clinging together against the dark, not our hope of getting things right. (p. 166)

Once again, this is not to suggest that truth is merely social, but rather to highlight that the claims people take to be true are, in a significant way, efforts that bring people together. This is helpful to consider the social function of the truths I hold in my own communities—as a clinician invested in the empirical sciences, as a citizen concerned about social welfare, and as an adult son attentive to the realities of my aging family. But it is also instructive to appreciate the truths other people live by in their own communities. Making sense of aging, dementia, and caregiving through pragmatism allows me to remain attuned to the way basic life experience can mean something different across time and place, and also to appreciate how people pursue meaningful lives and come together in this context. At once, pragmatism shows how basic life experience is constituted within cultural parameters, and reveals the human agency that underlies it. This is why listening to others matters and what, it is hoped, cultural competence might ultimately come to signify.

THE MORAL OF CAREGIVING

On the last day of fieldwork I came to visit Alex at his home. I wanted to again express gratitude for his invaluable support of the project and to reaffirm the friendship we had developed in the process. Alex's wife was completing finishing touches on a rug to be sold at their home, and his mother and grandmother returned from the market to see me off. Recalling my first visit, I was struck by his son, who had now begun to walk and even learned how to kick a soccer ball. Life seemed to be progressing, full of the milestones and excitement that older generations come to notice of younger ones.

During this visit Alex informed me that Cynthia, Carlos's wife with severe Alzheimer's, had recently passed. Alex had heard the news through his cousin, someone who was closer to Carlos's family than either of us. Only moments later, we heard a brass band parade through the street. The music was slow and somber. Deep horns and sonorous drums punctuated long silences. It was a juxtaposition to the jubilant sounds I had heard in the Danza and other festive occasions. It came from a distance, and slowly made progress toward the church. Alex told me this was Cynthia's funeral procession. I wondered how Carlos and his family experienced this loss—how his larger family and community had come together in this difficult moment. I thought about the obvious point that approaching caregiving as a social practice also implicitly posited how care was an expression of love and an anticipation of loss. And, amid these thoughts, I reflected about how this project put into focus the way being human is part and parcel of acknowledging one's own vulnerabilities and responding to others' in moments of need. Caregiving experience and practice might differ across time and place, but the core of both seemed to highlight the interdependency implicit to life itself.

In this moment of solidarity, I wanted to approach Carlos and his family to acknowledge the loss I suspected they felt. But I also intuited that they wanted to be alone, among themselves. They were cautious throughout most of my fieldwork about whether to invite me into their home, and then later about whether to continue talking to me about their caregiving experience. Throughout my time in Teotitlán, their hesitancy served as a continual reminder of the lack of *confianza* I was challenged to navigate, the way that all caregivers to some degree seemed to experience difficulty talking about this intimate dimension of their lives. And yet, despite their hesitancy, I came to know much about Carlos and other caregivers. At one point, Carlos explained his decision to invite Alex and me into their home, and the way it was situated in a desire to help other caregivers in the future. "Caregivers are the ones that have the hardest time," he said.

> So, that's why I would like that this investigation leads to a medicine or a remedy so this [experience] is rarer. Because not all elders have families that will have patience for them. And there are other elders that don't have relatives, or anyone at all. They must live like animals. I'm sure that's the way some people live. And there are people that only live two in a house. And those people can't do anything [for forgetful elders]. So I'm wishing the best for you [and this study]. And [I think] this is a good investigation.

Carlos did not know about Sophia being alone in caring for her husband, nor was he aware of Pablo and Vanessa, who cared for Maria even though she was not in their immediate family. But his comments spoke to an implicit solidarity with them and an understanding of community dynamics that directly shape the experience and meaning of care itself.

Through the testimony of voices woven together in this book, we not only have an intimate perspective of how life is maintained in moments of dependency, but also acquire a perspective of how specific values are upheld and regenerated in the process. In Teotitlán, we see how respect for elders is simultaneously upheld and challenged through signs of their forgetfulness, and how households come together to reaffirm and redefine what cohesion means in its wake. As others have noted before, caregiving reveals the importance of specific, local values. These values are embraced and pursued not through abstract reasoning about them, but in the concrete practices inherent in attending to dependent persons (Mol, Moser, & Pols, 2010). The caregivers in this study embodied this sort of practical, concrete wisdom.

Caregivers stand to teach us about the unavoidable reality of human dependency, and the varying ways we might come together to meaningfully respond to it. In a different work, Kleinman and Hanna (2008) write that caregivers are best understood as antiheroes, persons who do not engage in physical combat to change the world, but rather have an effect through subtly perturbing it. Indeed, the caregivers I had the opportunity to meet in Teotitlán exhibited similar attributes. They not only put into focus the ways local values and identity are maintained through social practices, but more importantly highlight the purpose and meaning of coming together to support others in need. Teotiteco caregivers are antiheroes by reminding their community about what is at stake in the context of the ambivalence that accompanies social change—and how neighbors might attend to this reality in order to reaffirm values that matter. Much to their nature as antiheroes, the caregivers studied in this book promote positive social change not through actively forcing it, but through personally embodying it. Their everyday isolation reveals the larger ambivalence and tension that marks social life in Teotitlán. And their commitments to care for elders express how they come to affirm and redefine local values in its wake. Through their near-imperceptible work—and the concomitant suffering inherent to it—caregivers are key figures in Teotitlán who effect change that matters.

As a guest to Teotitlán I recognize that I would be unfit to conclude with my own statements about how caregivers might impact the community. So, I turned to Alex to consider how his involvement has impacted him, how our partnership was not only useful for collecting information but also productive for occasioning social change. This was a theme we had discussed throughout our fieldwork, but it was most salient toward the end. We recalled challenges that we had faced and surprises we had encountered. We remembered the gratitude that caregivers expressed, despite some having been so reluctant to talk. Alex had helped me document others' voices so well, and so, in asking my questions, I explained that I wanted to also feature his own.

> ALEX: It's very different the way I see [things now]. . . . There are some people that need a lot of help, and I didn't realize that people needed [that much] help.
>
> JON: Why do you think you didn't realize it before?
>
> ALEX: Probably because I [spent so much time with] people who didn't [need] much help. . . . So, I was in this little bubble where everything was good around me. But now . . . my point of view [has] changed.

JON: So how do you think it has changed?

ALEX: Well, first of all, now that we've finished interviewing and we met a lot of people, now I would like to help those people. And not just old people, but also other people with [other] needs.

JON: Why do you think this whole experience made you want to do that?

ALEX: Because [I saw] the way they lived. . . . And that's something that [sparked] in me a desire to help. . . . [Now] I would like to help, and with nothing in exchange. Just do it as a part of me, as a part of my life.

Alex's words are expressive of the way he has been impacted by discovering the details of caregiving. In learning about a form of life he did not know existed—and encountering caregivers' suffering—he shows how caregivers do, in fact, subtly perturb and concretely enact change. His conviction to help "with nothing in exchange" is expressive of his larger desire to respond. It is expressive of him being a member of the community whose values are shaped and embodied by quiet heroes he now knows exist.

Alex's perspective is helpful for putting into focus how the observations made in this book might lead to broader, structural interventions and related health policy. His words are resonant precisely because they testify to caregivers' lived experience—precisely because, through learning about others' devotions to care, he has come to care as well. Through being a citizen of the community, he plans to reengage neighbors and help instill the type of understanding he knows they now lack. His lead provides suggestions for how others might follow suit. It is my hope that lessons drawn from this book might percolate to everyday awareness in Teotitlán to begin to mollify caregivers' isolation. Neighbors ought to know about a sector of the community that is facing difficulty so that they can come together to offer support and reaffirm cohesion. This, after all, is so much of what seems to define life in Teotitlán.

While efforts might be made toward addressing the local stigma of age-related forgetfulness or programmatically integrating forgetful elders and their caregivers back into the community, Alex's response illustrates that what matters most is that people are heard and understood. Thus, the lessons drawn in this book are not directly translatable to clinical intervention, nor do they suggest that a more sophisticated or informed campaign could dispel the pain experienced on a local level. Yes, these could help—but they are also not enough. Nor are there easy answers to deal with the nuanced dynamics and myriad tensions of contemporary life. Rather, the lessons drawn in this book help inform an overall sensibility in attending to people's isolation and responding to their possible suffering. For caregivers, as a means to foster dialogue among their neighbors, one possible response might involve hosting community meetings through 70 y Más, Prospera, or other existing programs. Another response might involve *tequio* or *cargo* services to provide additional social support to families that could benefit from it. But regardless of what concrete action one comes to take, caregivers teach that appropriate interventions are ones that meaningfully acknowledge individuals for their daily efforts. They are ones that honor caregivers' dedication to maintain a sense of cohesion within the parameters of contemporary life. That is why, however one decides to respond, this book's lessons do not lend themselves to a codified, scripted answer. Rather, this book teaches about the importance of opening oneself to listening in order to respond, to fostering engagement and conversation among members of one's community, and to locating a certain humility and pragmatism for those encountered outside.

Notes

PREFACE

1. Such categorizations are misleading because they tend to suggest an essentialized vision when people do not fit into neatly defined boxes. As I explain in the introduction, it is misleading to simply understand the community that is the subject of this book as "Zapotec" without attending to the nuanced ways this identity is defined. Moreover, such categorizations are problematic because they are complicit in reinstating power dynamics, what Edward Said (1978) calls the "politics of othering," the process of studying people's differences and, in so doing, asserting responsibility to educate or civilize them. As Denzin and Lincoln (2005) state on the first page of their book, research on other cultures is a "way of representing the dark-skinned Other to the white world" (p. 1). I approach both issues as a reminder to be cautious about how one ought to engage in cross-cultural research and remain sensitive to the claims made in the process. This sentiment is similarly expressed by James Clifford (1988), who writes that "while ethnographic writing cannot entirely escape the reductionist use of dichotomies and essences, it can at least struggle self-consciously to avoid portraying abstract, ahistorical 'others'" (p. 23). I hope this book stays true to this approach.

2. For greater discussion on culture as a dynamic, nonstatic category, see Kleinman and Benson (2006) as well as Kirmayer (2012).

3. For readers interested in larger epistemological issues concerning psychology's engagement with social constructionism, see Patricia Greenfield's (2000) essay on "What Psychology Can Do for Anthropology, or Why Anthropology Took Postmodernism on the Chin." Greenfield argues that psychology has avoided many of the "postmodern crises" that face anthropology concerning culture and objectivity because it has continued to frame itself as a scientific discipline that is distinct from an interpretive hermeneutic one. Whether or not one agrees with Greenfield's thought-provoking arguments, my turning to social constructionism concerns clinical issues about cultural difference, not epistemological ones that define psychology as an empirical science. Ultimately, this draws upon a distinction between psychology as a natural science and psychology as a human science. Both produce valid truths, but they aim to study different parts of human life. As Leswin Laubscher (2016) writes in defense of the latter, "A natural scientific psychology, with its experiments, statistics, and the guardrails of the scientific method, is seduced into a causal, external viewpoint on the person. But human beings operate in the realm of meaning, lived experience, and complex and complicated relationships. . . . Simply transporting the methods, procedures, and assumptions of the natural sciences . . . onto human beings runs the risk of missing what is human about human beings" (p. 61).

4. Moreover, the National Institute on Aging and the Alzheimer's Association have proposed significant changes from the 1984 diagnostic criteria that are largely still adhered to in most clinical settings (Albert et al., 2011). A new "preclinical" diagnostic stage of Alzheimer's based on the presence of biomarkers will lead to issuing diagnoses prior to the development of cognitive impairment. This diagnostic shift was initially intended to serve research purposes, but it has undoubtedly influenced clinical practice as well, leading to a larger number of diagnosed cases (Carrillo et al., 2013).

5. This is the basic principle of the recovery movement in clinical psychology. Recovery from psychiatric/psychological illness is not understood as the removal of all symptoms or all restoration of functioning, but rather as one's personal acceptance of and life in the context of those symptoms. Acceptance provides the ground for new possibilities of life-meaning and purpose (see Corrigan et al., 2007; Deegan, 2003). Other writers from phenomenological psychology further contribute to this perspective. Roger Brooke (2002) writes of Alzheimer's disease that "there is always a person first, and that person is using whatever cognitive and psychological resources he or she has to understand and deal with the disintegration of a world" (p. 138; see also Romanyshyn, 2012).

INTRODUCTION

1. This practice is what led Spanish chroniclers and some contemporary scholars to claim that the Zapotec religious system was polytheistic. Whitecotton (1977) writes that each community had a local patron deity and that Teotitlán was allotted *Xaquija,*

the Zapotec sun god, who was prominent in the Zapotec pantheon (p. 158). J. Marcus and Flannery (1996) contest this observation, arguing that "had the Spaniards [and contemporary scholars] described these heroic ancestors as 'saints' rather than 'gods,' they would have been closer to the mark" (J. Marcus & Flannery, 1996, p. 20). A more recent investigation led by Michael Lind (2015) argues that the Zapotec religion defies being understood through discrete Westernized religious constructs and that it likely featured an amalgamation of a pantheon of deities (including both gods and deified ancestors of the clouds), animatistic beliefs, and a hierarchal priesthood.

2. In other work (Yahalom, 2017) I explore the phenomenology of this encounter by engaging with the philosophy of Emmanuel Levinas.
3. For additional work on Teotitlán, see also: Cook and Binford (1990), Fitzsimmons (1972), Gagnier de Mendoza (2005). Hernández-Díaz (2012), Hernández-Díaz and Zafra (2007), Taylor (1960), and Vargas-Baron (1968).
4. Even the famed neurologist Oliver Sacks (2012) toured and devoted a book on Oaxaca's rich fern diversity.
5. Researchers note that the presence of inhabitants in Oaxaca's Central Valleys can be traced back as far as 10,000 B.C. with the region's earliest evidence of small communities of hunters and gatherers (J. Marcus & Flannery, 1996, p. 12; Smith, 1997). Other communities outside the Central Valleys existed in what is now the state of Oaxaca; yet Oaxaca Valley's irrigable and navigable land made it the de-facto capital of socioeconomic and political life. The most resounding image of the region's historical stature is Monte Albán, the former capital of the Zapotec empire and one of Mesoamerica's first cities—so celebrated by contemporary Mexican culture that the ancient ruins appear on Mexico's $20 peso note. Even today it is not difficult to gain a sense of Monte Albán's historical prestige and political might: the ruins are towering and expansive, resting on a mountaintop at the center where Oaxaca's three valleys come together, providing a stunning panoramic view.

Prior to the settlement of Monte Albán in 500 B.C., the Central Valleys were populated by more than eighty-five communities (J. Marcus & Flannery, 2000, p. 367). While these communities always continued to be inhabited during Monte Albán's sovereignty, they formed a regional alliance and coalesced power to fight against neighboring empires like the Mixtecs. Researchers note that this marked the birth of the Zapotec people, and Monte Albán as the religious, scientific, and political center in this region of Oaxaca. By 800 A.D. Monte Albán supported a population of more than 30,000 individuals—the largest political settlement in the southern Mexican highlands—and gained power over much of the region (Blanton, 1978).

While Monte Albán declined in 800 A.D., the scope and influence of the Zapotec empire can still be felt today. After its fall, for a five-hundred-year period that ended with the Aztec's conquest of Oaxaca in the fourteenth century, smaller empires competed for regional supremacy. Oaxaca was in a state of "balkanization" where no single power gained control, and different communities were able to develop autonomously (J. Marcus & Flannery, 1996, p. 394). This further contributed to the community-specific identities that continue to flourish today. See also: Oudijk, 2000.

6. To this end, Joseph Whitecotton (1992) argues that, although most research on Oaxaca refers to a unifying "Zapotec" ethnicity, this view is mistaken because there is nothing bounded or definitive about being Zapotec. Attempts to understand different communities as Zapotec derive from sixteenth-century Spanish chroniclers who projected their own sociocultural constructs of ethnicity and race onto indigenous populations (p. 64). Hence, challenging the claim that Oaxaca is home to sixteen indigenous groups, some have even argued that the number of different Oaxacan cultures more accurately reaches four thousand (Ordóñez, 2000).

7. Teotitecos also distinguish among *themselves* according to language use. There exists a grammatical difference between members who live in the more elevated, northern area of the community and those who reside below. This difference appears to be based solely on location, and does not correspond to socioeconomic categories.

   Beyond language practices, Teotitecos also distinguish themselves from neighboring communities in other ways—labor practices like weaving and production of religious wax candles, and preparation of local varieties of drinks like *atole* and foods like *tamales*. Public performances like *Lunes Santos* ("Holy Monday") and *La Danza de la Pluma* ("Feather Dance") are a further case in point. Performed in front of the church whose walls incorporate carved stones of Zapotec deities and patterns, *La Danza* is a two- to eight-hour performance by a select group of choreographed dancers clad in feathered headdresses and locally tailored clothing who recount the story of the fall of the Aztec empire and Teotitlán's reception of the Catholic doctrine (see Hernández-Díaz, 2012).

8. Since the colonial period, this system accounts for how a significant number of local communities have been able to maintain local control in governance. The *cargo* system may be traced back to two principal forms of colonial governance—civic cargos and religious *cofradías*—introduced by the Spaniards over Oaxaca's indigenous populations (Chance & Taylor, 1985). The first, civic cargos, was a system where select individuals held a series of increasingly prestigious government posts. In indigenous villages these positions were typically allotted to native rulers, circulating power among privileged persons, and also preserving traditional civic order (Murphy & Stepick, 1991, p. 18). Under this system, local rulers were held responsible to comply with the *encomienda* system, whereby villages were subjected to serve individual colonists, leading to exploitation and forced labor of the indigenous population (W. B. Taylor, 1979, p. 14). Colonists demanded that villagers produce specific products that were then bought at prices lower than market value, thereby "encouraging" villages to move beyond subsistence farming toward economic exchange. This also fostered the type of craft specialization inherent to many of Oaxaca's indigenous communities today.

The second form of governance was established through the Catholic Church, and its introduction of cofradías (confraternities or religious corporations). After Pope Alexander VI ruled that Spain had the religious sovereignty to conquer the New World, Conquistadores were given the dual mission of both seizing land for the Spanish Crown and evangelizing indigenous populations. The Dominicans were Oaxaca's first missionary order to arrive in 1528 (seven years after Oaxaca capitulated to the Spaniards) and Teotitlán was officially evangelized in 1580 (Gagnier de Mendoza, 2005, p. 114). The Church's efforts were largely carried out through cofradías that were established in regional centers. Cofradías were religious institutions that collectively owned and managed land and livestock, and sponsored elaborate community-wide celebrations of patron saints. Indigenous populations were converted to Catholicism, but the decentralized organization of the cofradia system allowed Catholicism to be adapted within the customs of a given community, and thus gave rise to the stark "unorthodoxy" found in contemporary Mexican Catholicism.

9. Technically, one representative from every married couple or household is required to provide service.

10. For more on Teotitlán's cargo system, including analysis of the history of its structure and religious-civic division and how elders' roles have begun to change within it, see Stephen, 2005 (pp. 231–243).

11. After Mexico gained independence in 1810, politicians were ambitious to create a nation of citizens united under the same laws, religious values, and aspirations for industrial growth. Prior to this period the Catholic Church controlled the majority of civic and public life. This changed during the mid-nineteenth century, with the federal government insisting on the separation of church and state, taking control of religious property. Yet the drive toward economic and cultural development also fomented a national image of the indigenous "Indian" as an obstacle, in need of being appropriated within national culture. The sentiment ruptured after the Revolution of 1910 with almost obsessive preoccupation in creating a new nationalism that sought to *"mestizo-ize"* (whiten) the indigenous population. These ambitions perpetuated racist ideologies and exerted pressure for indigenous communities to engage in the national workforce. *Indigenismo* was a core feature of revolutionary and postrevolutionary ideology, centering on an idea of Mexican national identity that romanticized indigenous culture as the origin of Mexico, while, in so doing, creating a construct of the "Indian" as a figure of the past at odds with modernity (Lewis, 2006). Indigenismo respected indigenous communities' autonomy for self-governance, while simultaneously aiming to integrate and "modernize" them into the nation (Knight, 1990). Such emphasis undoubtedly impacted Oaxaca's indigenous communities.

12. The 1994 Zapatista uprising in Chiapas is perhaps the most known example of social unrest against this trend. The uprising protested NAFTA's implementation and used it as a crystalizing image of indigenous peoples' marginalization at the expense of national efforts to engage the international market.

13. For an early and still relevant study of how locals adapt and embrace tourism and related folkloric images of Mexican heritage, see MacCannell, 1984.

14. Yet as Stephen (2005) and Wood (2008) note, not all rugs are representative of traditional Zapotec culture. Teotitecos adapt to the demands of the tourist market, and many of their products also feature Navajo and other popular designs. This is another expression of the global influences in local culture.

15. Teotitlán's dual identity has existed for decades. As Lynn Stephen (2005) writes, since Mexico's early twentieth-century efforts to promote tourism by celebrating (caricatured) images of indigenous heritage, Teotitecos capitalized by "work[ing] self-consciously to maintain an aura of mystique about the community, reproducing stereotypes of indigenous artisans . . . creat[ing] a picture of simple precapitalist relations" (p. 33).

16. In contrast to common accounts of migration that appeal to a binary set of factors—"push" (owing to economic hardship in sending countries) and "pull" (owing to economic promise in receiving countries)—Teotitecos are best understood as migrating because of a complex set of reasons that mutually impact the other. Seth Holmes (2013) describes another Oaxacan community's experience of migration as a "forced movement for survival" that attends to the complexity of this decision-making process (p. 186). Teotiteco migration can similarly be understood in this light.

17. Oaxacan migration began during the years preceding the Mexican Revolution when individuals sought refuge from fighting, and expanded during the U.S. *bracero* programs that welcomed Mexican migrant workers during the 1910s and again in the 1940s to satisfy labor shortages caused by both World Wars (J. Cohen, 2004, pp. 54–56). Teotitecos participated in both *braceros* but achieved greater mobility to move back-and-forth in 1986 with the U.S. Immigration Reform and Act that gave migrants the legal opportunity to have permanent residency (J. Fox & Rivera-Salgado, 2004, p. 6; Stephen, 2007, pp. 11–12). Today, Teotiteco and other indigenous migrants have continued to move in pursuit of economic opportunity, giving rise to what Charles Hale (2002) calls the "extraordinary mobilization of indigenous people" (p. 485). More than 60 percent of Oaxacan households in the Central Valleys have at least one member living in the United States (J. Cohen, 2004, p. 6). And, despite Oaxaca's small size and distance from the U.S. border, Oaxacan migrants account for 4 percent of total U.S. migrant population (J. Cohen, 2004, p. 20).

18. Yet many of Oaxaca's indigenous migrants continue to face discrimination once in the United States. Though my acquaintances in Teotitlán reported having positive experiences in the United States, many migrants from Oaxaca are unable to speak Spanish and are discriminated against not only by host country residents, but also by other Mexican migrants as indicated by terms like "*Oaxaquitas*" (little Oaxacans) and "*Indios sucios*" (dirty Indians) (J. Fox & Rivera-Salgado, 2004, pp. 11–12). This is vividly articulated in Seth Holmes's recent work (2013), where he describes how

"marginalization begets marginalization" through the way that indigenous Oaxacan farmworkers are subject to greater discrimination than other migrant workers precisely because they are indigenous (p. 78).

19. With half of Oaxaca's population living in communities of fewer than 2,500 people (INEGI, 2014), many communities face the real threat of becoming a *pueblo fantasma* (ghost town). There is greater burden on remaining residents to uphold endangered local forms of governance and religious customs; families and communities struggle to maintain a sense of cohesion; and local economies become dependent on remittances (J. Cohen, 2004, pp. 111–123; Worthen, 2015). Migration also carries ramifications for the psychological well-being of those who remain and return. For example, Whitney Duncan's (2012, 2018) study on Oaxaca's mental health industry shows that clinical practice is flourishing, in part, as a response to the pervasiveness of migration and associated psychosocial trauma.

20. Many Teotiteco migrants cross the border legally, having received temporary visas, work permits, or citizenship through the *bracero* program during the 1980s. Yet for those who do not have legal documentation, life is considerably more difficult as families are rendered apart and individuals face grave economic and physical risks crossing the border. Many researchers (Abrego, 2014, Holmes, 2013, Yarris, 2017) have explored the humanitarian impacts of this aspect of migrant life.

21. At least originally, as Raymond Williams (1977) reminds us, the word "culture" was used as a noun to describe process: the culture *of* something, like crops, animals, or minds (p. 13). Today our working definition is different. Culture not just as a set of prescriptive norms (e.g., something one must do in order to be part of the culture), but rather an orientation people adopt to their social world that draws upon "shared-in-common resources" (Holstein & Gubrium, 2012, p. 163). This idea is similar to what Clifford Geertz (1973) calls the "webs" of meaning inherent to a group of people (p. 5). Yet Williams reminds us that despite these semantic shifts, culture was and remains a dynamic construct that always is a work-in-progress. As explained in the main body of the text, I adopt Williams's sense of culture in this book.

22. Teotitlán is referred to in Zapotec as *Xigie*, which translates to mean "enchanted" and "below the stones," referring to a prominent rock perched above the community that some hold to possess divine powers.

23. After Eric Hobsbawm's (2012) study of "the invention of tradition"—the way that some customs that are purported to be rooted in distant history are actually more recent cultural inventions—sociologists like Anthony Giddens (2002) have gone so far to observe that all traditions are invented. Again, the point is that tradition is not anchored to a specific moment in history, but rather situated in broader social change.

24. Thinking of caregiving as an instance of "reproduction" also implicitly invokes ideas about fertility. Feminist scholars have rightly called attention to the way that this notion of caregiving highlights its reality of being undervalued labor in capitalistic

societies that link personhood with productivity and practices of care as forgotten forms of labor (Busch, 2015; Glenn, 2010; Wilkinson & Kleinman, 2016).

25. Social constructionism has been criticized since Bruno Latour's (2007) critique on disciplines that presuppose the "social" as a type of material that differs from other phenomena. Latour argues that it is erroneous to posit that something like a social realm can be mobilized to explain world phenomena when it is precisely how aging exists socially that sociologists must pursue. While I agree with Latour on theoretical grounds, I continue to reference work in the social sciences for the way they help analyze interpersonal practices like caregiving and social representations like aging and illness.

26. Anthropologist Johannes Fabian (2006) also makes a similar allegation that researchers in his field are liable to overlook the cultural differences that they orient themselves to study. "The failure of anthropological discourse," he writes, "has been a failure to recognize the epistemological significance of alterity" (p. 178). Fabian is talking about anthropology's tendency to acquire information about other people's differences, while leveling those differences into a preconceived framework of understanding.

27. More recent scholars in pragmatism have varying perspectives of this idea. Richard Rorty (1979) defends an extreme antirealism perspective on pragmatism through his social-practice approach to truth. According to Rorty, all knowledge derives from social practice, and it is erroneous to believe that anything can be taken to represent a "mirror" to underlying objective nature (see also White, 2009). Other pragmatic philosophers like Jurgen Habermas (2000) and John McDowell (2000) critique Rorty's extreme antirealism and defend a commonsensical realism that, they differently argue, must be implicit in knowledge claims. Though I am aware of these debates, engaging with these philosophical subtleties is a distraction from pragmatism as I use it in this book, as a means to attend to truth's *function* in social life and to establish a clinical gaze that is attentive to cultural varieties of illness.

28. Cultural pragmatism is an attempt to address clinical tendencies that conceptualize "culture" in a decontexutalized, static manner. It contributes to the list of alternative approaches to studying culture, responding to Laurence Kirmayer's (2012) call for additional metaphors to better inform clinical practice. Presenting cultural comptence as a instance of humility was originally articlated by Tervalon and Murray-Garcia (1998). These authors rightly distinguish between "comptence," a term that implies a mastery of a finite body of knowledge, with "humility," a sensibility that promotes self-reflection, check of power imbalances, and mutual respect (see also Hook et al., 2003). This adds to other metaphors of cultural competence, including "cultural responsiveness" (Sue et al., 1991) and "cultural safety" (Papps & Ramsden, 1996). And, more recently, "structural competency" (Metzl & Hansen, 2014), which emphasizes awareness of social structures to appreciate how varying social conditions cause and contribute to health disparities. Each of these approaches helps address the

growing need for clinicians and social scientists to adopt alternative perspectives when attempting to address the role of culture.

29. The phenomenologist J. H. van den Berg (1985) explained: "Most essential in phenomenology is that the nature and the characteristics of human existence are to be found not by investigating man's subjectivity, but by studying and describing his world" (p. 8). Phenomenology, as a method, derives from the work of Edmund Husserl (1900/1970) who is known for his motto, "We must go back to the things themselves" (p. 252). He argued that human inquiry must attend to the specific lifeworld of various individuals. Amedeo Giorgi (1970) was one of the first to apply phenomenology to contemporary psychological research. In other work (Yahalom, 2013), I address the history of phenomenology and its application to psychological inquiry.

30. In Teotitlán, many Zapotec speakers use an abbreviated version of the Spanish word—*confianz*—to refer to *confianza*. However, *relilaz* is another Zapotec word that refers to this concept, literally translating to mean that one has a "straight heart." This issue is further illustrated through neighboring language practices. Although Teotitlán's Zapotec does not feature it, other Zapotec communities make a grammatical distinction in first-person plural pronouns, between "we-including-you" and "we-not-including-you." This is yet another illustration of how much identity in Oaxaca is formulated on the local level.

31. Typically, when researchers approach a field site they are viewed in terms of social categories salient to that community (Harrington, 2003, p. 607). No doubt, the mixture of warmth and restraint I was given was a result of this reality; I was initially perceived to be a consumer, like the countless other tourists who visit Teotitlán interested in buying rugs. Challenging this perspective was not easy and took considerable time. Through the quotidian conversations—with people in the market, vendors on the street, and other passersby—I drew upon affiliations like shared experiences in California, distinguished myself through my identity as a psychologist, and expressed intent to document the community so that its needs might better be met.

32. Further, this draws on Clifford's (1986) understanding of culture as a set of relational practices, illustrating how "to think of a cultural poetics that is an interplay of voices" (p. 12). As I will come to discuss, this interplay not only involves exchanges between Alex and me as co-researchers, but also between Alex and Teotiteco caregivers as members of the same community.

33. In Zapotec there is a distinction about what one forgets. *Rienlá'az* refers to the forgetfulness of objects, whereas *raguenlá'az* is the forgetting of a person. As I will explain in the subsequent chapter, inquiring about the latter implied greater stigma.

34. Moreover, I reasoned that my former training in geriatric psychology would assist me to differentiate among dementias. So, instead of following Byron Good's (1992)

recommendation to medical anthropologists to stay focused on diagnostic categories and submit them to cross-cultural research, I would first study the symptoms as they manifested locally, and *then* apply my training to make sense of what was occurring diagnostically. To be sure, I am aware that differentiating between the dementias is difficult and cannot be adequately done without rigorous neuropsychological testing. My main concern was to differentiate between progressive dementias (like Alzheimer's disease or Lewy Body Dementia) and dementias stemming from injury (like strokes in vascular dementia); the former are "progressive" in the sense that they involve gradual memory loss, whereas the latter involve abrupt changes from which one may recover. This is a critical distinction that I maintain throughout the book.

35. Alex was central to this strategy. He waited for me to ask basic questions in Spanish and English and subsequently held in-depth conversations with groups of households about their opinions.

36. For an interesting discussion that is an exception to this claim, see Stephen, 2005, p. 209.

37. To facilitate comparative analysis of data across interviews, I created an interactive computer spreadsheet where I inputted more than four hundred excerpts of text categorized by code, theme, and household. This spreadsheet was my primary way to access data yet, again, I continued to return to study field notes and original transcripts for greater context.

38. *Pláticas* (chats) are informational presentations that provide bio-psycho-social information that are required of elders if they are to receive their monthly pension through 70 y Más, the government-sponsored program designed to provide financial support to elders living in poverty. They similarly exist for Prospera, another pension program that serves the broader community.

39. Because I did not initially know whether I would succeed in gaining access in Teotitlán, I adopted a strategy similar to Loïc Wacquant (2011) and followed Alzheimer's disease and dementia wherever I suspected it might appear, tracing its circulation through different contexts and among different social actors. In Oaxaca City, my fieldwork extended to include interviews with directors at each of Oaxaca's two government-funded *casas de hogar* (nursing homes), professional and family caregivers for elders with dementia, psychologists, psychiatrists, and other persons invested in geriatric care. I interviewed medical residents and a *curandera* from a different Zapotec community. I visited other pueblos in the state and volunteered for an NGO that provides bio-psycho-social support for elders in extreme poverty. I studied newspapers, collected informational pamphlets, and attended a conference focused on geriatric care. Though these experiences are not the focus of this book, they were significant in developing my understanding of Oaxacans' broader perception of aging and dementia.

40. This approach also helped resolve underlying epistemological tensions within qualitative research theory. One of the biggest paradoxes is the way in which interviews are at once understood to arrive at the subjective or personal experience of participants, while they are also known to be shaped by the event of interviewing. In other words, the problem is that researchers often mistake language as a direct channel that transmits undiluted information about the speaker's experience. Yet some contend that language is more accurately understood as a joint production between speakers (Suchman & Jordan, 1990; see also Crapanzano, 1992). As Packer (2010) writes, "the interviewee's subjectivity [and what is expressed during the interview] is an *effect* of the . . . interview, not a preexisting, independent personal experience that is the content expressed in what is said" (p. 99). Conducting focus group interviews with households helped provide an answer to this perspective of language by instead studying the negotiation of meaning *among* social actors, not their private experience.

41. See: Behar, 1996; Denzin & Lincoln, 2005; Fabian, 2014; Fine, 2017; Lyons et al., 2013; Mies, 1983; Riessman, 2002; Said, 1978; Wilkinson & Kleinman, 2016.

CHAPTER 1. THE PROBLEM OF AGING IN TEOTITLÁN

1. Unless otherwise noted through the use of full names, throughout this book all names and identifying information have been changed to protect confidentiality.

2. Duncan's (2018) work on "psy-sociality" advances insight about social dynamics in Oaxaca, tracing the emergence of new forms of social life based on Euro-American ideas about psychology and mental health. In contrast to local notions of personhood, these groups have fomented alternative understandings based on personal growth and self-actualization, and have subsequently led to novel ways for individuals to come together in the context of social change.

3. Of course, individuals can act independently. But these orientations rather help situate the context in which individual acts are decided upon, highlighting how broader social concerns orient everyday experience (see Royce, 2011, p. 2; Stephen, 2005, p. 209). People can earn money for their own individual gain, jettison family obligations after migrating, and pursue other, individualistic lifestyles. But the point is that broader social spheres continue to orient how people experience everyday decisions, including the provision of care for elders. At the very least, *not* fulfilling such expectations is something that people are aware they are overlooking.

4. To further illustrate how households are primary, in Teotitlán the onus to fulfill cargos does not fall on specific individuals so much as on the household. Married couples are expected to live in their own homes and contribute through one representative from this unit to provide cargo service. This also helps navigate the complicated issue of how residents living abroad are able to fulfill cargos and *tequios* (volunteered labor for short-term projects); the household represents their contribution.

5. In contrast to English, where the verb "to care" simultaneously refers to practice (care for) and sentiment (care about), the Zapotec of Teotitlán has two different words for each meaning. To refer to the practice of care, the verb *ruinlau* is used as in the sentence, *"Ruinlaua xmama"* (I care *for* my grandmother). To refer to the sentiment of care, the verb *rikiela'z* is used as in the sentence, *"Rikielaza xmama"* (I care *about* my grandmother). This is but one answer to the empirical question raised by Buch (2015) regarding whether other non-English languages bridge affect and practice in a single verb.

6. Nija'nu A.C. is a Mexican nonprofit organization supporting elders in the Mixtec region that live in poverty with little or no family support. The organization aims to address immediate needs, such as hunger and unsafe living conditions for elders living in Santo Domingo Tonalá, as well as serving surrounding communities. Readers can find out more at http://www.nijanu.org.

7. Throughout Oaxaca, these gendered divisions of labor are changing in the context of globalization and related systemic trends. For interesting discussions on how women in Oaxacan indigenous communities have become empowered and responded to these changes, see Andrews (2014) and Worthen (2015).

8. The same image was also displayed on a printed banner inside the municipal building. Instead of a hand-painted depiction, this version was a computer graphic. The origins of the image are not known. As the case with most public campaigns, this mural is in Spanish. Zapotec is primarily a spoken language and rarely written.

9. This trend is not exclusive to Mexico, but mirrors worldwide statistics, where improving longevity rates are also equally unprecedented: by 2050 the number of older persons (over 60) will exceed the number of young (under 18) for the first time in world history (United Nations, 2002, p. xxviii).

10. All subsequent demographic information was acquired through individual review of data provided by Mexico's census bureau, Instituto Nacional de Estadística y Geografía (INEGI, 2005).

11. This trend is consistent across the state of Oaxaca, despite the fact that Oaxaca had one of Mexico's lowest life expectancy averages of 72.5 years in 2013 (INEGI, 2015).

12. Social constructionism simultaneously points attention to how meanings of growing old have been taken for granted, and also implicitly states that the current issues facing aging populations (such as financial problems facing retirement, social isolation, etc.) could otherwise be different (see Hacking, 1999, p. 6).

13. Within gerontology, social constructionism has been at the center of major theoretical and clinical transitions. Instead of prescribing the correct or "healthy" way for elders to age, gerontologists have historically turned to social constructionism to describe how the aging process is inherently multifarious and contingent upon social factors and contexts. They argued that old age is a social construct that varies across cultures

and historical periods (Achenbaum, 2005). Social constructionism was first applied to study aging during the 1970s when gerontologists sought theoretical justification to respond to two dominant perspectives in the sociology of aging (e.g., see Carroll Estes, 1979; Gubrium, 1972; Harris, 1975). First, gerontologists sought to contest Cumming and Henry's (1961) disengagement theory, which posited that the individual and society mutually prepare for separation in anticipation of death, such that the aging individual gradually becomes further disengaged from society. This view not only suggested that social disengagement is typical for elders, but that disengagement *ought* to occur during the aging process. Although disengagement theory is no longer popular among contemporary gerontologists—it perpetuates ageist stereotypes rather than ameliorates them (Butler, 1975)—many public institutions like United States' Medicare and the Mexican pension system (70 y Más) are founded upon it (with a rationale that the government ought to provide assistance to elders who are presumed unable to provide for themselves). Later, gerontologists turned to social constructionism as a response against Rowe and Kahn's (1987, 1997) successful aging theory, which argued that elders are capable of aging "successfully"—defined by avoidance of disease and disability, maintenance of physical and mental capacities, and engagement in life. This theory was originally intended to be a positive alternative to past gerontological theories, but it carried the concomitant burden of establishing an ideal of healthy aging that proved, for many, to be unattainable (Holstein & Minkler, 2007, pp. 15–16). Through this theoretical approach, aging and the features associated with it—senility, dependency, and physical debilitation—became understood as a relational process, not something that elders undergo irrespective of their social surroundings (Cole & Ray, 2010; Gergen, 2009). In this way social constructionism offered a means to challenge the tendency to reduce aging to an individual problem, inviting consideration of how surrounding social settings were not only contextualizing the problems faced by elders, but also complicit in perpetuating them. And, through it, gerontologists have mobilized social constructionism to raise awareness about implicit ageist assumptions (Butler, 1975), to improve social policy designed for elders (Bernard & Scharf, 2007; Estes, 2001), and to inform caregiving practices to meet psychosocial needs of elders (Kitwood, 1997; Sabat & Harré, 1992).

14. This information is available from the work of Juan de Córdova, a sixteenth-century Spanish Dominican linguist who studied the Zapotec language in Teotitlán and is famous for producing one of the first dictionaries to help study Mexican indigenous languages. The significant difference between colonial and contemporary Zapotec is an illustration of the evolution of this primarily verbal (nonwritten) language. Other evidence of this evolution will be seen through this book via Zapotec words that have incorporated Spanish cognates.

15. In addition to this semantic distinction, there exists a third type of person who has authority based on wisdom and experience. The *tsïgul* (Zapotec original, often

referred to as *huehuete*, a Nahuatl word) is typically an elder who is hired to adjudicate proper adherence of local traditions. For example, the tsïgul often presides over wedding and engagement rituals, as when a women's family is asked for permission to marry through an elaborate and prolonged affair. The tsïgul is distinct from the representative family member (*bengul* or *bingul*) who gives advice to married couples at the wedding ceremony.

16. The Spanish original is gender-specific and uses the feminine pronoun (*ella*) to refer to individuals that have Alzheimer's disease. This provides additional insight to how Alzheimer's disease is represented as a disease that primarily impacts women.

17. This again invokes Rabinow's (1996) concept of biosociality. Whereas above I presented this term as a form of sociality within the public sphere, it also is useful to explain the sociality inherent between medical providers and the larger public. In part, this relationship could be understood as an instance of commodifying vital life processes (like senility and death), and the subsequent emergence of novel biosocial truths that serve specific capitalistic ends. As Gibbon and Novas (2008) so pointedly write, "life itself has become economically valuable" (p. 12; see also Rose, 2007).

18. Aside from newspapers, Lundbeck, an international pharmaceutical company, published the only other public document I had encountered that promoted awareness of Alzheimer's disease. The document is titled "Patient Care for Alzheimer's Disease" [*Cuidados del paciente con Enfermedad de Alzheimer*]. In interesting rhetoric that appeared more pertinent to U.S. settings than Mexican ones, it contrasts "autonomous and independent" elders from individuals with Alzheimer's disease. "A large majority of elders are autonomous and independent and a minority demand care. This is the case of people who suffer from Alzheimer's disease" (translation mine). Focus on elders' autonomy is a striking contrast from the way in which elders are locally seen as being part of larger social networks. This is a further illustration of Duncan's (2018) point on "psy-sociality," the process by which novel ideas about psychology and selfhood circulate through the growing influence of the mental health industry.

19. Moreover, among the three psychiatric hospitals in Oaxaca, none view dementia as a psychiatric condition that would fit within the parameters of their care. Of course there are exceptions, but I was told that elders are expected to be situated within their own sources of support. Should an elder with dementia arrive to one of these facilities without support, one resident psychologist told me, that elder would eventually be forced to live on the street.

20. This diagnostic entity has existed in Mexico since the late eighteenth century, when Mexican doctors first began to embrace French biomedicine over humoral theory. Historian of Mexican medicine Germán Somolinos D'Ardois (1976) locates the first professional use of the term "dementia" to a document written on July 29 in 1775 by three medical Mexican doctors (trained in France) who were considering the case of an old professor who had developed curious behavioral and cognitive symptoms.

Although the exact symptoms are not known, what is of interest is the way the three doctors directed their attention, debated over etiology, and, in so doing, introduced a new category of illness to local medical practice. Somolinos D'Ardois (1976) writes: "What is instructive of their opinion for the medical historian interested in Mexican psychiatry . . . can be found [in the adjudicators'] words . . . [compared to] those [words] used . . . centuries earlier. They keep talking about sadness and melancholy, [but here] the word "dementia" [appears for the first time] and also the concept of mania" (p. 109, translation mine). It is not clear how this term initially made an impact on local medical practice, yet today's use of the diagnostic category demonstrates the importance of this event.

21. These symptoms have remained the defining feature of Alzheimer's disease and account for the progression of clinical symptoms. Amyloid plaques and neurofibrillary tangles are known to first impair subcortical regions, including the hippocampus (responsible for memory-formation), and then spread to neocortical regions. This physiological progression accounts for the course of Alzheimer's disease symptoms: difficulty remembering new information and depression are common early symptoms; confusion, disorganized thinking and judgment, and inappropriate behavior are moderate symptoms; difficulty with basic motor tasks (including speaking, swallowing and walking), and seizures are found at the advanced stage. Alzheimer's disease also increases susceptibility for pneumonia and other infections, indirectly leading to death.

22. In part, this began to change through the efforts of Robert Butler (1975), who argued against what he termed "ageism," which he claimed was inherent in the idea that senility is a typical feature of aging. It also changed through the political campaign led by Robert Katzman, who was one of the strongest political voices to claim that age of onset should be eliminated as a criterion because Alzheimer's disease and senile dementia (e.g., "normal" senility among elders) were, in fact, neurologically the same entity. Katzman's successful campaign significantly increased the number of Alzheimer's disease cases in the general population, and challenged the assumption of inevitable cognitive decline associated with old age (Fox, 1989, p. 73). This argument, combined with subsequent public awareness programs led by the Alzheimer's Disease and Related Disorders Association (now known as the Alzheimer's Association), transformed Alzheimer's disease into one of the most popular and devastating epidemics (for further review of this history see Ballenger, 2006).

This history gave rise to the popular representations surrounding Alzheimer's disease found throughout U.S. settings today. As of 2014 it is estimated that one in nine older persons suffer from Alzheimer's disease, with the majority (82 percent) aged seventy-five or older (Hebert, Weuve, Scherr, & Evans, 2013). The prevalence of Alzheimer's disease increases with age such that persons younger than 65 years are estimated to have a 4 percent risk; those between 65 and 74 years carry a 15 percent risk; people between 75 and 84 years carry a 44 percent risk; and, for those who age beyond 85 years, the risk reduces to 38 percent ("2014 Alzheimer's disease facts and figures," 2014; Hebert et al., 2013). These numbers are projected to increase in severity such that, by 2025 when the majority of baby boomers reach age 65-plus years, Alzheimer's disease is expected to be prevalent in 7.1 million Americans, a 40 percent increase from 2010 (Hebert et al., 2013).

23. Further, the purported objectivity of scientific inquiry has been called into question. Researchers have argued that scientific tools like fMRI are a form of "cultural activity" whose findings are not an objective mirror of nature because they draw upon statistical assumptions and perspectives that are, in themselves, rooted in a specific cultural outlook (Choudhury, Nagel, & Slaby, 2009; Margulies, 2012).

24. Appreciating the role of culture also puts in perspective how mental processes are themselves shaped and influenced by broader sociocultural forms. This was originally documented by the pioneering neuropsychiatrist Alexander Luria during his research on different industrialized parts of Uzbekistan, showing how perception and understanding are shaped by social conditions (Nell, 1999).

25. Once again, the study of Alzheimer's as a phenomenon situated in and shaped by local factors does not suggest "misappropriation" of biomedicine. Surrounding culture inextricably shapes clinical understanding, such that one cannot conduct a study on mental health without attending to surrounding sociocultural horizons (Kleinman, 1980, 1988a). As demonstrated in the contested history of Alzheimer's disease within U.S. settings, the interpretation of what is "normal" versus "pathological" has consistently been shaped by cultural beliefs. This is not an exception in mental health fields, but the norm: the implicit knowledge that we draw upon to discern illness comes from cultural perspectives, not objective frameworks. In this vein, all psychological-psychiatric systems are said to be "ethnopsychiatric," constructed within "cultural tapestries" that shape the definition and meaning of illness (Gaines, 1992, p. 8).

This suggests not only that meanings of Alzheimer's differ across time and space, but that those meanings carry inherent clues to the dynamics of the setting in which they arise (Henderson & Henderson, 2002; Henderson & Traphagan, 2005). All medical systems are open and malleable, such that new medical concepts are regularly introduced and medical knowledge is continually adapting to surrounding social discourses (Good, 1994; Leslie, 1980; Lock & Nichter, 2002). Leveraging these insights helps explain how psychiatric concepts like Alzheimer's are taken from one setting and introduced into another.

CHAPTER 2. IDIOMS OF DISTRESS

1. Although rarely mentioned in the literature, pragmatism is a cornerstone of Nichter's original focus on the communicative functionality of idioms of distress—what he

at times refers to as a "transactional approach"—and also when he cites the work of semotician Charles Morris (1971) for providing a theory of language that attends to how communication carries concrete impact on social life (Nichter, 2010, p. 403, note 8). Inspired by the fact that Nichter explicitly references pragmatism in his early work, the subsequent analysis shows that returning to this philosophical origin helps account for why studying idioms of distress matters, and how maintaining a philosophically coherent framework puts into focus not only the "metaphoricity" of how idioms are communicative of—and embedded within—cultural parameters (Kirmayer, 1994), but also the social functions that such metaphors serve. Pragmatism is an important theoretical development in Nichter's conception of idioms of distress because it allows for the appreciation of cultural difference as a matter of social function, while being grounded in a view of truth that does not succumb to assessing the purportedly "objective" validity of cultural difference. In other words, pragmatism attends to the truth of idioms of distress insofar as truth is understood to serve a function in everyday life.

2. This type of questioning shifts attention away from an "objective" neo-Kraepelinian approach (i.e., a focus on symptomology and overlooking what underlies symptoms), toward appreciating how illness expressions "serve adaptive functions" that engage in social life by communicating social or personal distress (Nichter, 2010, p. 402). This approach has produced a burst of global research regarding the social anxiety expressed in psychological and medical distress, (Abramowitz, 2010; Yarris, 2017), the indicators of psychopathology across cultures (Lewis-Fernández et al., 2009, Hinton et al., 2010), the clinical utility of developing culturally sensitive assessment measures (Guarnaccia et al., 2003; Hinton et al., 2012; Kaiser et al., 2013; Kohrt et al., 2013), the understanding of variances in help-seeking behavior (Hinton & Lewis-Fernández, 2010), to name but a few topics.

3. Davidson states that this notion is indebted to philosopher W. V. Quine. I refer to it as Davidson's principle because I was not able to locate its origins and because Davidson is often credited for it.

4. Medical pluralism was first studied by Charles Leslie (1980) who, by demonstrating the existence of multiple medical systems in most societies, argued that traditional medicine continues to be relevant and that biomedicine is rarely hegemonic (see also Good, 2010). More recently, as Lock and Nichter (2002) articulate, research in medical pluralism has revealed the vast range of medical practices that exist across and within the same cultures. It also provides a perspective to examine how traditional medical systems have responded to biomedicine, creating an alternative medical viewpoint to "modern" medicine's association with industrialization, capitalization, and other forms of global engagement (Comaroff, 1981).

5. As I will discuss in greater detail in the following chapter, I am aware of the inherent difficulties using the term "belief" to discuss people's perspectives of health conditions

(see Good, 1996). Yet I deliberately use this term not only because it is the best translation for how caregivers described certain opinions about medicine and underlying etiology, but also because it situates the implicit power-dynamics when it is compared to caregivers' "knowledge" about medicine.

6. In addition to traditional and biomedicine, Oaxaca is also home to homeopathic medicine (see Finkler, 2001b; Hunt, 1992; Whiteford, 1995) and Euro-American psychological perspectives (see Duncan, 2017a, 2017b, 2018). My decision to not include these in my framing of etiological understandings of forgetfulness is because homeopathy and psychology did not seem directly relevant to how caregivers were conceptualizing its cause.

7. For a more detailed discussion of how traditional medicine is constituted by broader social factors, see Menéndez, 1994.

8. Pre-Hispanic Zapotec religious practice was based on what Whitecotton (1977) calls a "quid pro quo principle" where individuals paid tribute to receive favor, and believed that ignoring divine commands would result in punishment (p. 165). The Zapotecs further distinguished between animate and inanimate matter, the former possessing vital force that was worshipped through ritual (J. Marcus & Flannery, 1996, p. 19).

    Moreover, the Aztecs, who likely had an influence on Zapotec culture after their conquest of Oaxaca, believed in a world of supernatural and divine forces of dual principles—day and night, birth and death, good and evil—whose continual struggle led to cosmological harmony (Belsasso, 1969, p. 32; see also Ortiz, Davis, & McNeill, 2008, pp. 277–280). To this end, the understanding of the self was rooted in a dynamic equilibrium, captured in the Aztec term *ixtli-in yollutl*, which literally translates to "face-heart." Mesoamerican cultures believed that the individual was born "faceless," symbolically lacking a distinct self and, through moral education, developed a unique face that could be presented to the community (Padilla & De Snyder, 1988). In contrast to Western metaphysics, Mesoamerican culture did not have a distinct notion of soul (Somolinos d'Ardois, 1973, p. 69). The closest concept was *tonalli*, a notion to describe the individual personality as it is constituted through dual forces of the moon and the heat of the sun (Beltrán, 1978).

9. Prior to the Spanish conquest, psychiatric illnesses in Aztec culture were conceptualized as manifesting from a general condition termed *yollopoliubqui*, which translates from Nahuatl to mean "that which has left the heart" (Somolinos d'Ardois, 1976, p. 27). This condition referred to a type of emotional disturbance that would be similar to what today is meant by the term "going crazy" or "losing one's head" (Padilla & De Snyder, 1988, p. 62). There were four basic etiologies said to cause illness: pathology owing to natural order, pathology owing to enemy's curses, divine punishment, and loss of self owing to supernatural forces (Somolinos d'Ardois, 1973, pp. 68–70). These four etiologies were expression of broader disequilibrium of cosmic forces, and illness was a concern for the entire community (Somolinos d'Ardois, 1973, p. 25; 1976, p.

19). Treatment was provided by a trained and respected physician—*tonalpouqui*—who prescribed treatment according to a highly developed taxonomy of medicinal plants, exorcisms, trephination, and talk therapy in effort to reestablish equilibrium (Padilla & De Snyder, 1988, pp. 62–63).

10. The medicine brought by the Conquistadors was predominantly Greek (Galenic, to be specific) and conceptualized health and illness according to the equilibrium of four humors—fire, air, water, and earth. Treatment was based on the "principle of opposites" where deficit humors were supplemented, or ones in excess were reduced (Hernández Sáenz & Foster, 2001, p. 20). This remained the dominant medical system in Mexico until the introduction of biomedicine in the mid-nineteenth century.

11. My turn to these traditional conceptions of illness is not to suggest an essentialized reading of Teotitlán. It would be foolhardy to argue that the following traditional concepts involve the same undiluted pre-Hispanic metaphysics. Instead of suggesting that these notions somehow represents a "traditional" understanding of forgetfulness, I present them to suggest a more nuanced point regarding medical pluralism and the way Teotitlán is entrenched within a complex syncretic landscape. Etiologies are not traditional *or* biomedical, but rather situated within a pragmatic mode of understanding, constituted by the mutual existence of both. Here, a traditional understanding of soul loss is leveraged to explain age-related forgetfulness, a purportedly new, "modern" illness. This helps demonstrate how traditional ideas continue to have relevance as new, biomedical ones are encountered—while avoiding the claim that traditional medical ideas somehow contest, eclipse, or succumb to new ones. Though this is a subtle point, I consider it important because it avoids the type of essentialist arguments that view settings like Teotitlán as living apart from or resisting "modern" medical ideas.

12. The Zapotec expression used, *bian anim* (soul loss), further sheds light on what type of soul is lost—it is the soul that departs from the deceased (in comparison to *garlien*, which refers to the soul of living persons). While soul loss is presented as a "traditional illness category," the concept more accurately illustrates how traditional ideas fuse with nontraditional ones. As discussed above, Mesoamerican pre-Hispanic culture did not believe in a "soul," but rather tonalli, a conception of the self that was based upon ecological harmony with different forces of the physical world. The person was constituted within and by his or her location, and, as such, personhood was not an abstract entity that transcended the surrounding environment (Belsasso, 1969, p. 32; Beltrán, 1978, 1992). As a Catholic community, Teotitecos *do* believe in the soul and consider it liable of being lost. Hence, the equation of *bianan* with *pérdida del alma* highlights Mexico's syncretic cultural tradition, coalescing pre-Hispanic understanding of the self as constituted through surrounding nature, the European notion of a transcendent soul, and even an African understanding of selfhood as constituted by one's shadow (Somolinos d'Ardois, 1973, p. 70).

13. An illustration of treating soul loss is provided in chapter 5.

14. This understanding is an inversion of common views held in U.S. settings where depression is viewed as a comorbid symptom of Alzheimer's disease. However, it is interesting to note that there is evidence that history of depression is known to be associated with increased risk of Alzheimer's disease (Mourao, Mansur, Malloy-Diniz, Castro Costa, & Diniz, 2016; Ownby, Crocco, Acevedo, John, & Loewenstein, 2006).

15. This case further contextualizes research on the epidemiology of depression in Mexican settings. Slone et al. (2006) found that, while the prevalence of depression in Mexico was lower than that known in the United States, its symptomology was different. Mexican symptoms of depression were primarily somatic in nature, involving fewer cognitive features like worthlessness and guilt. Among caregivers, feelings of worthlessness and rumination described by caregivers of their elders suggest how cognitive features of depression can be experienced with greater force, such that they are used to explain forgetfulness itself.

16. There were additional etiologies that other caregivers used to account for age-related forgetfulness. These included (1) physical injury to the brain and (2) poor diet. I do not feature these in the main chapter because they were exclusively used by caregivers to explain vascular (not progressive) dementia. The only exception was Sergio, Manuel, and Linda, who considered a past head injury to the elder's brain as a possible cause of his forgetfulness.

17. Much effort is directed toward combating this opinion within the United States. For example, in the first pages of *The 36-Hour Day* (2011), the most popular guide written for dementia caregivers, the authors explicitly state that "severe memory loss is *never* a normal part of growing older" (p. 7). As I have discussed, this debate stood as the foreground of whether Alzheimer's disease constituted an actual disease at the time of its discovery (see chapter 1).

18. Moscovici's (2000) discussion of "cognitive polyphasia" is particularly relevant here for the way it accounts for how the same individuals are able to maintain multiple understandings from epistemologically different (and conflicting) perspectives (p. 241).

19. The idea of mental faculties as dependent on finite wet resources has a long history that extends to ancient Greek humoral theory. Galen hypothesized that the lifecycle is determined by a process of perpetual drying: the infant is endowed with moisture, compared to the old person, who is dried out (see Cole, 1992, p. 8). Considering how Spanish Conquistadores introduced Galenic medicine to Mexico, it is not surprising that these two concepts are so similar across time and space. Elsewhere in Mexico, Young and Garro (1993) present a related understanding of the lifecycle based on the concept of *fuerza* (literally, "force" or "strength") that eventually becomes used as the individual ages (p. 46).

CHAPTER 3. HEALTH-SEEKING BEHAVIOR

1. At the time of fieldwork, the monthly pension elders received from 70 y Más was $580 pesos (approximately $35 U.S.).

2. Adapting Kleinman's (1980) framework for conceptualizing types of medical providers, in Teotitlán I view health-seeking behavior as occurring within the following overlapping sectors: the popular sector involves home remedies; the folk sector is comprised of curanderas (traditional healers who possess specialized spiritual and local knowledge); and the professional sector consists of medical doctors, nurses, and other specialists whose practice is locally sanctioned and politically legitimized (p. 50). In this way, my use of the term "folk" is not diminutive, but rather meant to point to the common ways of acquiring knowledge. Gaines' (1992) use of "folk" psychiatry is an example (p. 5). Or, in a similar vein, Norget's (2006) use of the term "popular" refers to the ambivalent and contradictory beliefs inherent to laypersons (p. 16). Like Norget, my use of the term "folk" refers to a perspective distinct from elite medical practice. Folk knowledge is common, widely dispersed, and part of everyday life.

3. I am aware that representing people's views about medicine as a matter of "belief" is delegitimizing and authorizes one's power as observer (Good, 1996, p. 20). Yet in this chapter I continue to use the word "belief" to account for people's (dis)engagements with traditional medicine because, as I will come to show, this concept (and its juxtaposition to statements about "knowledge" of biomedicine) best accounts for how and why individuals justify their health-seeking behaviors.

4. While it is commonly written that the Conquistadores introduced humoral theory, anthropologists like Alfredo López Austin (1988) contest this claim by arguing that pre-Hispanic indigenous societies actually held their own version similar to humoral theory. This theoretical debate is interesting, but for the purpose of this chapter, I adopt the more standard understanding that humoral theory originates from the Spanish Conquest.

   Again, "other abroad sources" refers to those concepts of illness (e.g., the evil eye) brought from Spanish, Muslim, and Jewish Conquistadores, as well as African slaves. The Spanish Conquistadores were a heterogeneous group that did not introduce a single coherent medical system, but rather brought multiple and conflicting ones.

5. I refer to curanderas in the feminine form because all practicing folk healers I encountered in Teotitlán were women. Yet there exist many male curanderos throughout Oaxaca, Mexico, and Latin America. In Teotitlán, curanderas do not typically rely on medical practice as a primary means of income. Most have other professions and practice traditional medicine on the side.

6. I initially found this to be contradictory. I reasoned that either *susto* was viewed as the cause of all these other illnesses, or there was inconstancy in the profession.

As my fieldwork developed I learned to not resolve this dilemma. I came to realize that traditional medical practice operates on a different logic than my own, with greater suppleness than I was accustomed to, given the specialization I had known of medical practice in the United States. As Good (1996) notes, biomedical practice operates with a distinct hermeneutic that is primarily oriented toward diagnosis. Other medical systems like traditional perspectives in Oaxaca are less concerned with differentiating symptoms and illness types, and instead focused on establishing personal and ecological harmony.

7. In Zapotec this diction is also present, but carries additional sophisticated differences in comparison to other verbs. The Zapotec verb "to know with certainty," *nanna*, is used in sentences like *"Nanna kety raku xbii,"* which translates to mean "I know that you do not have a cold." The Zapotec verb "to think something is the case," *rizak*, is used in sentences like *"Txa rizaka ziab nisgie,"* which translates to mean "I think it will rain." While *rinii* is a Zapotec word to refer to "knowledge," one would not use it to refer to make a sentence like "the doctor knows I am sick." Instead, a Zapotec speaker would attribute this information to the authority of the doctor him/herself, as in sentences like *"Doctor gunii na yuu dxabaa,"* which translates to mean "The doctor told me I am sick."

8. Curanderas might encourage individuals to seek allopathic help, but that physicians rarely refer to traditional specialists complicates Stacy Pigg's (1995) notion of "harmonious pluralism," which she describes of settings where "many kinds of healing are not seen as different systems. . . . [Rather] [t]hey merely constitute what is understood to be an open set of locally available options" (p. 23).

9. However, it is rumored that Cortes wrote to King Charles V to not send Spanish doctors because indigenous medics were more than competent (Hernández Sáenz & Foster, 2001, p. 22). Whether or not the anecdote is true, it reflects the highly developed medical tradition that existed prior to the Spaniard's arrival. Further, it shows how even the Conquistadores found value in local culture and healing practices.

10. There are good reasons that Carlos and his family visited a neurologist and not a general medical doctor, but to protect their privacy, I am intentionally omitting this facet of their story.

11. Medical visits are free for elders on the state pension program, and are subsidized to twenty pesos for those who pay out of pocket.

12. In addition to pension programs, Mexico's universal health-care coverage also expands the scope of biomedical influence. Though highly disputed, Mexico today claims to have reached universal health-care coverage with a complicated three-tiered insurance industry. All individuals in the formal economy are guaranteed health coverage through either IMSS (social security for workers in the private sector) or ISSSTE (for state workers). Though these programs provide coverage for approximately

half of Mexican citizens, they are not as important in serving Teotitlán because its residents are mainly a part of the informal economy. The third insurance program enacted in 2003, the Seguro Popular, is designed to cover individuals not part of the formal workforce, who are more economically disadvantaged compared to the rest of the national population. Though this program has dramatically increased enrollment, critics have argued that it does not guarantee access to quality care, or ensure that healthcare services are utilized among poorer populations (Gutiérrez, 2014).

13. The way caregivers prioritized elders' desires to not seek medical care (over their own curiosities about whether doctors might be able to help) was also expressed during meetings with other caregivers as well. Yet along with households like Sergio's, who chose to not consult doctors, I was surprised that many households perceived me as a representative of biomedical practice and inquired whether I might be able to help them. Hence, while some households chose not leave home and pursue medical help, they are receptive to that help if it comes to them.

14. I also recognize that this may be an instance of collusion. Returning to a theme from the previous chapter, Sergio's fidelity to his father's opinion makes sense given his desire to minimize the significance of forgetfulness. It colludes with Sergio's desire to continue life as normal, to believe that his father's memory lapses are no reason for concern.

15. This point also touches on what Kitwood (1997) calls the "Alzheimerization of dementia," the way in which symptoms of dementia are increasingly viewed through notions about Alzheimer's disease in the United States and other biomedically oriented settings (p. 22).

CHAPTER 4. RELATIONSHIPS WITH ELDERS

1. Studying lived experience has been a cornerstone of phenomenological research since Dilthey (1887/1996), and is traced through Husserl (1900/1970) and Merleau-Ponty (1945/1962) and appears in nearly all related contemporary work. It refers to the prereflective dimensions of human existence—what it is like to live through something (van Manen, 2004). This concept is consistent with my engagement with anthropology's concept of subjectivity, but I choose to emphasize the later because it applies greater focus on the social factors that constitute experience.

2. Research shows that caregiver burden is experienced differently across cultures. Latino and other minority caregivers in the United States tend to experience less symptoms of depression and stress compared to Caucasian cohorts (Connell & Gibson, 1997; yet for an interesting exception, see Harwood et al., 1998).

3. Some threads within the research canon acknowledge this point. For example, Monin and Schulz (2009) rightly suggest that family caregivers experience difficulty not only

because of the physical demands of their roles, but also because they are dealing with concrete issues about death and dying. To conceptualize this point, Monin and Schulz introduce the idea of "emotional contagion," a process whereby caregivers experience suffering because they are exposed to the suffering of another person, not merely because of the physical demands of their labor (p. 12). They argue that psychological support aimed to address the interpersonal realm of caregiving experience is critical to meeting their needs. Arguments like this are vital in moving beyond an idea of caregiving as merely a realm of physical adversities. While caregiving is demanding for many reasons, its fundamental interpersonal nature is what makes those demands meaningful and resonant.

4. Although I assume that caregiving also leads to conflicts among caregivers themselves, I did not come across instances to support this. One reason likely owes to the nature in which I collected my data. Meeting with the entire household helped foster insight into how meaning is negotiated among household members, but it also limited the extent to which individuals could discuss how other members caused difficulties.

5. One way to account for this apparent paradox is to note that caregivers view forgetfulness as normal and, as a consequence, attributed blame to the elders' personality, not their illness. This resonates with studies on Mexican American families who similarly attribute caregiving difficulties to personality changes (Berkman et al., 2005; Drumond-Andrade, 2012, p. 188). This attribution further carries ramifications for how caregivers relate to elders.

6. This helps contextualize observations made in chapter 2 about how attributing forgetfulness to sadness helps caregivers pragmatically respond. Further, Pablo and Vanessa's description of learning about Maria's diagnosis touches on an historical debate about whether diagnosing elders improves or worsens how they are perceived and treated. Those who believe that diagnoses help have defended their arguments through attribution theory, a perspective that views diagnoses like Alzheimer's as allowing families to decrease blame of the elder, develop greater patience, and increase sympathy (see Wadley & Haley, 2001; Weiner, 1993). In contrast, others appeal to Erving Goffman's (1961) labeling theory that views dementia diagnoses as leading to negative consequences that stigmatize and shame the elder (see Kitwood, 1997; Sabat & Harré, 1992). As Pablo and Vanessa's case illustrates, diagnosis enacts both positive and negative consequences, such that the two perspectives cannot easily be separated. This highlights the complicated nature of the debate between attribution and labeling theories, but demonstrates how both are relevant and helpful toward understanding how biomedical ideas impact and foment new forms of relating to elders.

7. As anthropologists have long argued, death is not an objective biological event, but an experience whose meaning varies widely from one context to another. For example, Lock's (1997) cross-cultural study of different definitions of death across

the United States and Japan demonstrates how underlying values generate vastly different responses to death and dying.

8. This local function stands in contrast to U.S. settings, where comparing forgetful elders to children adds greater stress to caregivers and stands for a symbol of deteriorating relationships. As I will discuss in more detail, this is perhaps one reason why there exists such strong domestic effort to challenge this perspective.

9. Comparing elders to children might also invoke a deeper metaphysical perspective about the nature of the soul. For example, compared to deceased adults who are believed to be required to repent for their sins in purgatory, in Oaxaca when children die they are believed to be *angelitos* (little angels) and permitted direct access to heaven (Norget, 2006, pp. 118–121). They are exempt because they are not capable of sinning; they lack awareness to have had behaved differently. In contrast to the melancholic music that accompanies pallbearers at funerals of deceased adults, when children die the music is bright and upbeat. Relatives are expected to be cheerful because of knowledge that children have direct access to heaven. Of course, this does not mean that families are not distraught at the loss of children; I came across families who experienced the death of the child with a profound sense of loss. In this way, comparing elders to children may help view elders as not being accountable for their actions. It helps caregivers understand that elders are not intentionally being difficult, and that it is likely not worth the effort to try to get them to change.

10. Rautman's notion is based on psychoanalytic theory, postulating that the envy and resentment that characterizes children's relationships with their parents eventually becomes fulfilled through the aging process. Adult children consequently experience shame by witnessing the enactment of their fantasies.

11. Also making sense of caregiving through this perspective, Richard Schulz's (2000) caregiving handbook describes role reversal as a common experience of caregiving, yet one that has the potential to cause resentment and anger toward the dependent elder, threatening to compromise provision of care (p. 41).

12. This was not only true in Teotitlán but also consistent with my broader fieldwork. For example, in Oaxaca City one friend who happened to be a caregiver for her mother diagnosed with Alzheimer's told me that this is the most difficult aspect of caring. She recalled her mother as being strong and strict up until a few years ago, but now felt unmoored as she witnessed her mother's confusion, tearfulness, and insecurity. At one point this caregiver confided to me and said, "It's hard to remember who my mother really is."

13. As discussed in the introduction, the distinction between two different types of souls helps shed further light on how the dying process is locally understood. Dominga's comments could perhaps be understood as a chronologically reversed instance of the dying process. Here, Dominga appears to suggest that her uncle's *anim* (the soul

that departs when one dies) has already separated from his body, while *garlieng* (the soul one has while living) keeps him physically alive.

14. Only two exceptions appeared. The first was Carlos's family, the caregiver whose wife was diagnosed with Alzheimer's after a finger amputation. Perhaps the severity of his wife's condition—and the way attempting to manage her behavior no longer seemed to be an option—Carlos said he and his family do not view his wife as a child. The second exception was in my interview with Luis and Laura, the caregivers who recently moved in to live with Laura's mother, who showed signs of mild forgetfulness. While they did not explicitly say Laura's mother was like a child, at one point Laura said, while discussing their frequent arguments, that while Laura continues to view her mother as a mother, she is not sure about how her own mother views her. Quoting Laura, "I think she's the one who has forgotten who is her daughter."

CHAPTER 5. RELATIONSHIPS WITH THE COMMUNITY

1. There also exist two non-Spanish Zapotec cognates to refer to responsibility, yet these are rarely used among younger generations. *Zagunilà'àz* is an adjective used to describe a person who is dependable, attentive to others, and responsible for commitments made. Deriving from the word Zapotec word for "heart," *la'z*, this adjective is a part of the group of Zapotec words that describe inner convictions or personal experience (e.g., *relilaz* means to have faith, *rikiela'z* means to worry, *redxula'z* means to enjoy). The second Zapotec word to describe responsibility is *nia* and translates to mean "to look after or care for someone." For example, elders are heard saying *"Tu nia naa"* (Who will care for me?). Alex and the majority of participants used neither word, and referred to responsibility through *responsabl*, the Spanish cognate.

2. This is what gerontologists refer to as the "generational contract," where one generation invests care in another with the implicit expectation that they will be cared for when it is needed. Though Mario and other caregivers expressed uncertainty whether such contracts will be fulfilled—that is, whether future generations will care for them—this situation is not unique to Teotitlán and has been noted across cultural spaces and epochs, even depicted in the Jewish Bible (see Bengtson & Achenbaum, 1993).

3. I received contradicting information about the costs of nursing homes. Employees told me that they were free to residents, while others in the mental health industry said that this is a misrepresentation, and that residents are required to make payments that render such services unaffordable to many.

4. Moreover, Carlos and Francisco also doubt that a professional caregiver would be able to care for Cynthia as well as they do. Implicit is this stance is the idea that the person best suited to provide care for Cynthia is the one that cares for her the most—and, because Carlos and Francisco want what is best, they consider themselves responsible. In Francisco's words, he personally wants to provide care for his mother

because he knows that he would regret losing time should someone else assume the responsibility.

5. Despite the common ways caregivers compared forgetful elders to children, they did not believe elders' souls were the same as children. Like all other adults, forgetful elders have sinned during their lifetimes, and they are expected to similarly repent.

6. Stephen's (2005) study in Teotitlán similarly talks about the prevalence of gossip at various moments. For example, at one telling point she features the story of a woman weaver who became the subject of community gossip, eventually ruining her planned marriage (p. 315). Vignettes like this further speak to gossip's local prevalence and strength. For more on gossip in southern Mexican rural communities, see Browner (1986) for an interesting case study on women who are described as being caught between desire to have fewer children and social pressure (through gossip) to be prolific.

7. The dynamics of this exchange are further interesting for the way Manuel and his family tries to manage Alex's and my own opinion about Pedro's perceived mistreatment. Linda asserts that she *does* uphold the responsibilities that people gossip about: she tells her husband to change his clothes, and later her family descriptively illustrates other acts of care. I take these statements as her efforts to prove to Alex and me that gossip about her is not true.

8. Levinas often describes this encounter with otherness in terms of destitution—suffering—which singles-out the subject to respond. Levinas (1969/1992) writes, "To recognize the Other is to recognize a hunger. To recognize the Other is to give" (p. 75). Levinas argues that this event is the "pre-original" grounds of subjectivity (1974/1998b, p. 10). Pre-original because one cannot make sense of an event before responsibility, and is thus the event that leads to human subjectivity: the other's call singles-out and summons the subject to be ethical, to be something above an animal fulfilling basic needs, and hence birthed into a human subject. I further develop this phenomenology and consider its application to caregiving in a separate article (Yahalom, 2017).

9. Many researchers have made a call to move research from limited, academic inquiry to a matter of critical, social justice. See: Behar, 1996; Denzin & Lincoln, 2005; Fabian, 2014; Fine, 2017; Lyons et al., 2013; Mies, 1983; Riessman, 2002; Said, 1978; Wilkinson & Kleinman, 2016.

EPILOGUE

1. There also exists a Zapotec word, *dgul*, which literally means "elders," but in this context also refers to the *fiesta* of elders. For more detail on the event, see Gagnier de Mendoza (2005), who provides the only known published description of this event in Teotitlán. While the *Danza de los Viejos* is part of local tradition, it is more popularly celebrated in the Mexican state of Michoacán (see Hellier, 2001).

2. *Viejito* is a diminutive of the word *viejo*. Although literally translated to mean "little elder," many Spanish words in diminutive form do not literally refer to size, but rather express affection.

3. These men dressed as women also provide clues about homoerotic phobias. They know they will be groped by other dancers, and playfully joke about their discomfort. The community, in response, laughs and sanctions the gestures. Yet gay men who participate in the dance are subject to local gossip.

References

Abramowitz, S. A. (2010). Trauma and humanitarian translation in Liberia: The tale of open mole. *Culture, Medicine, and Psychiatry, 34*(2), 353–379.

Abrego, L. J. (2014). *Sacrificing families: Navigating laws, labor, and love across borders.* Stanford, CA: Stanford University Press.

Achenbaum, W. A. (2005). Ageing and changing: International historical perspectives on ageing. In M. L. Johnson, V. L. Bengtson, P. Coleman, & T. Kirkwood (Eds.), *The Cambridge handbook of age and ageing* (pp. 21–29). Cambridge, UK: Cambridge University Press.

Adelman, R. D., Tmanova, L. L., Delgado, D., Dion, S., & Lachs, M. S. (2014). Caregiver burden: A clinical review. *JAMA, 311*(10), 1052–1060.

Albert, M. S., DeKosky, S. T., Dickson, D., Dubois, B., Feldman, H. H., Fox, N. C., . . . Petersen, R. C. (2011). The diagnosis of mild cognitive impairment due to Alzheimer's disease: Recommendations from the National Institute on Aging-Alzheimer's Association workgroups on diagnostic guidelines for Alzheimer's disease. *Alzheimer's & Dementia, 7*(3), 270–279.

Alzheimer's Association. (2014). Alzheimer's disease facts and figures. *Alzheimer's & Dementia, 10*(2), e47–e92.

American Psychiatric Association (APA). (2013). *Diagnostic and statistical manual of mental disorders* (5th ed.). Washington, DC: American Psychiatric Association.

American Psychological Association (APA). (2017). Multicultural Guidelines: An Ecological Approach to Context, Identity, and Intersectionality. http://www.apa.org/about/policy/multicultural-guidelines.pdf.

Andrews, A. (2014). Women's political engagement in a Mexican sending community: Migration as crisis and the struggle to sustain an alternative. *Gender & Society, 28*(4), 583–608.

Apesoa-Varano, E. C., Barker, J. C., & Hinton, L. (2012). Mexican-American families and dementia: An exploration of "work" in response to dementia-related aggressive behavior. In J. L. Angel, F. Torres-Gil, & K. Markides (Eds.), *Aging, health, and longevity in the Mexican-origin population* (pp. 277–291). New York, NY: Springer.

Argáez-López, N., Wacher, N. H., Kumate-Rodríguez, J., Cruz, M., Talavera, J., Rivera-Arce, E., & Lozoya, X. (2003). The use of complementary and alternative medicine therapies in type 2 diabetic patients in Mexico. *Diabetes Care, 26*(8), 2470–2471.

Arnault, D. S., & Shimabukuro, S. (2012). The clinical ethnographic interview: A user-friendly guide to the cultural formulation of distress and help seeking. *Transcultural Psychiatry, 49*(2), 302–322.

Austin, A. L. (1988). *The human body and ideology concepts of the ancient Nahuas.* Salt Lake City, UT: University of Utah Press.

Austin, J. L. (1975). *How to do things with words.* Oxford, UK: Oxford University Press.

Ayalon, L., & Huyck, M. H. (2002). Latino caregivers of relatives with Alzheimer's disease. *Clinical Gerontologist, 24*(3–4), 93–106.

Ayora-Diaz, S. I. (1998). Globalization, rationality and medicine: Local medicine's struggle for recognition in Highland Chiapas, Mexico. *Urban Anthropology and Studies of Cultural Systems and World Economic Development, 27*(2), 165–195.

Baldassar, L., Baldock, C. V., & Wilding, R. (2007). *Families caring across borders: Migration, ageing and transnational caregiving.* New York, NY: Palgrave.

Baldassar, L., & Merla, L. (2013). *Transnational families, migration and the circulation of care: Understanding mobility and absence in family life.* New York, NY: Routledge.

Ballenger, J. F. (2006). *Self, senility, and Alzheimer's disease in modern America: A history.* Baltimore, MD: Johns Hopkins University Press.

Baxter, P. T. W., & Almagor, U. (1978). *Age, generation and time: Some features of East African age organizations.* New York, NY: Palgrave.

Behar, R. (1996). *The vulnerable observer: Anthropology that breaks your heart.* Boston, MA: Beacon Press.

Behnke, A. O., MacDermid, S. M., Coltrane, S. L., Parke, R. D., Duffy, S., & Widaman, K. F. (2008). Family cohesion in the lives of Mexican American and European American parents. *Journal of Marriage and Family, 70*(4), 1045–1059.

Belsasso, G. (1969). The history of psychiatry in Mexico. *Hospital & Community Psychiatry, 20*(11), 342–344.

Beltrán, G. A. (1978). *La medicina indígena*. Mexico City, Mexico: Universidad Nacional autonoma de Mexico, Instituto de investigaciones antropologicas.

Beltrán, G. A. (1992). *Medicina y magia: El proceso de aculturación en la estructura colonial*. Mexico City, Mexico: Fondo de Cultura Económica.

Bengtson, V. L., & Achenbaum, W. A. (1993). *The changing contract across generations*. New Brunswick, NJ: Transaction Publishers.

Berger, P. L., & Luckmann, T. (1967). *The social construction of reality: A treatise in the sociology of knowledge*. New York, NY: Anchor.

Berkman, C. S., Guarnaccia, P. J., Diaz, N., Badger, L. W., & Kennedy, G. J. (2005). Concepts of mental health and mental illness in older hispanics. *Journal of Immigrant & Refugee Services*, 3(1–2), 59–85.

Bernard, M., & Scharf, T. (2007). *Critical perspectives on ageing societies*. Bristol, UK: Policy Press.

Beyene, Y., Becker, G., & Mayen, N. (2002). Perception of aging and sense of well-being among Latino elderly. *Journal of Cross-Cultural Gerontology*, 17(2), 155–172.

Biehl, J., Good, B., & Kleinman, A. (Eds.). (2007). *Subjectivity: Ethnographic investigations*. Berkeley, CA: University of California Press.

Blanton, R. E. (1978). *Monte Albán: Settlement patterns at the ancient Zapotec capital*. San Diego, CA: Academic Press.

Braun, K. L., & Browne, C. V. (1998). Perceptions of dementia, caregiving, and help seeking among Asian and Pacific Islander Americans. *Health & Social Work*, 23(4), 262–274.

Brody, E. M. (1985). Parent care as a normative family stress. *Gerontologist*, 25(1), 19–29.

Brody, E. M. (1990). Role reversal: An inaccurate and destructive concept. *Journal of Gerontological Social Work*, 15(1–2), 15–22.

Brooke, R. (2002). Humanistic sensibilities in the assessment of dementia patients. *Humanistic Psychologist*, 30(1–2), 136–149.

Browner, C. H. (1986). The politics of reproduction in a Mexican village. *Journal of Women in Culture and Society*, 11(4), 710–724.

Bryceson, D., & Vuorela, U. (2003). *The transnational family: New European frontiers and global networks*. New York, NY: Bloomsbury Academic.

Buch, E. D. (2015). Anthropology of aging and care. *Annual Review of Anthropology*, 44, 277–293.

Buch, E. D. (2013). Senses of care: Embodying inequality and sustaining personhood in the home care of older adults in Chicago. *American Ethnologist*, 40(4), 637–650.

Calzada, E. J., Tamis-LeMonda, C. S., & Yoshikawa, H. (2013). Familismo in Mexican and Dominican families from low-income, urban communities. *Journal of Family Issues*, 34(12), 1696–1724.

Carey, M. A., & Smith, M. W. (1994). Capturing the group effect in focus groups: A special concern in analysis. *Qualitative Health Research*, 4(1), 123–127.

Carrillo, M. C., Dean, R. A., Nicolas, F., Miller, D. S., Berman, R., Khachaturian, Z., . . . Knopman, D. (2013). Revisiting the framework of the National Institute on Aging-Alzheimer's Association diagnostic criteria. *Alzheimer's & Dementia, 9*(5), 594–601.

Cervantes, J. M. (2008). What is indigenous about being indigenous? The Mestiza/o experience. In B. W. McNeil & J. M. Cervantes (Eds.), *Latina/o healing practices. Mestizo and indigenous perspectives* (pp. 3–28). New York, NY: Routledge.

Chance, J. K., & Taylor, W. B. (1985). Cofradías and cargos: An historical perspective on the Mesoamerican civil-religious hierarchy. *American Ethnologist, 12*(1), 1–26.

Chavela, R., Silvia. (2014, August 29). Detectan 20 casos de Alzheimer en el año. NOTICIAS, pp. 15A.

Choudhury, S., Nagel, S. K., & Slaby, J. (2009). Critical neuroscience: Linking neuroscience and society through critical practice. *BioSocieties, 4*(1), 61–77.

Clifford, J. (1988). *The predicament of culture.* Cambridge, MA: Harvard University Press.

Clifford, J., & Marcus, G. (2010). *Writing culture: The poetics and politics of ethnography.* Berkeley, CA: University of California Press.

Cohen, J. H. (2004). *The culture of migration in southern Mexico.* Austin, TX: University of Texas Press.

Cohen, J. H., Gijón-Cruz, A. S., Reyes-Morales, R. G., & Chick, G. (2003). Understanding transnational processes: Modeling migration outcomes in the central valleys of Oaxaca, Mexico. *Field Methods, 15*(4), 366–385.

Cohen, L. (1998). *No aging in India: Alzheimer's, the bad family, and other modern things.* Berkeley, CA: University of California Press.

Cole, J., & Durham, D. L. (Eds.). (2007). *Generations and globalization: Youth, age, and family in the new world economy.* Bloomington, IN: Indiana University Press.

Cole, T. R. (1992). *The journey of life: A cultural history of aging in America.* Cambridge, UK: Cambridge University Press.

Cole, T. R., & Ray, R. E. (2010). The humanistic study of aging past and present, or why gerontology still needs interpretive inquiry. In T. Cole, R. Ray, & R. Kastenbaum (Eds.), *A guide to humanistic studies in aging: What does it mean to grow old* (pp. 1–31). Baltimore, MD: Johns Hopkins University Press.

Comaroff, J. (1981). Healing and cultural transformation: The Tswana of Southern Africa. *Social Science & Medicine. Part B: Medical Anthropology, 15*(3), 367–378.

CONEVAL. (2012). Pobreza y rezago social: Indicadores de pobreza, Oaxaca 2010. Mexico City, Mexico: Consejo Nacional de Evaluación de la Politica de Desarrollo Social.

CONEVAL. (2016). Porcentaje, número de personas y carencias promedio por indicador de pobreza, Oaxaca, 2010–2016. https://www.coneval.org.mx/coordinacion/entidades /Oaxaca/PublishingImages/Oaxaca_cuadr01.JPG.

Connell, C. M., & Gibson, G. D. (1997). Racial, ethnic, and cultural differences in dementia caregiving: Review and analysis. *Gerontologist, 37*(3), 355–364.

Connor, L. (2001). Healing powers in contemporary Asia. In L. Connor & G. Samuel (Eds.), *Healing powers and modernity: Traditional medicine, shamanism, and science in Asian societies* (pp. 3–21). Westport, CT: Greenwood Publishing Group.

Cook, S., & Binford, L. (1990). *Obliging need: Petty rural industry in Mexican capitalism*. Austin, TX: University of Texas Press.

Corrigan, P. W., Angell, B., Davidson, L., Marcus, S. C., Salzer, M. S., Kottsieper, P., . . . & Stanhope, V. (2012). From adherence to self-determination: Evolution of a treatment paradigm for people with serious mental illnesses. *Psychiatric Services, 63*(2), 169–173.

Cox, K. K., Higginbotham, J. B., & Burton, J. (1976). Applications of focus group interviews in marketing. *Journal of Marketing, 40*(1), 77–80.

Crapanzano, V. (1992). *Hermes' dilemma and Hamlet's desire: On the epistemology of interpretation*. Cambridge, MA: Harvard University Press.

Cruz-Manjarrez, A. (2013). *Zapotecs on the move: Cultural, social, and political processes in transnational perspective*. New Brunswick, NJ: Rutgers University Press.

Cumming, E., & Henry, W. E. (1961). *Growing old, the process of disengagement*. New York, NY: Basic Books.

Cummings, C. H. (2002). Risking corn, risking culture. *World Watch, 15*(6), 9–19.

Das, V., Kleinman, A., Lock, M., Ramphele, M., & Reynolds, P. (Eds.). (2001). *Remaking a world: Violence, social suffering, and recovery*. Berkeley, CA: University of California Press.

Das, V., Kleinman, A., Ramphele, M., & Reynolds, P. (Eds.). (2000). *Violence and subjectivity*. Berkeley, CA: University of California Press.

Davidson, D. (1984). *Inquiries into truth and interpretation*. Oxford, UK: Oxford University Press.

Deegan, G. (2003). Discovering recovery. *Psychiatric Rehabilitation Journal, 26*(4), 368.

Denzin, N. & Lincoln, Y. (2005). The discipline and practice of qualitative research. In Denzin, N. & Lincoln, Y. (Eds.), *The SAGE handbook of qualitative research* (3rd ed., pp. 1–43). Thousand Oaks, CA: Sage.

Dewey, J. (1998). *The essential Dewey: Pragmatism, education, democracy* (L. Hickman & T. M. Alexander, eds.). Bloomington, IN: Indiana University Press.

Dillman, R. (2000). Alzheimer disease: Epistemological lessons from history. In P. J. Whitehouse, K. Maurer, & J. F. Ballenger (Eds.), *Concepts of Alzheimer disease: Biological, clinical and cultural perspectives* (pp. 129–157). Baltimore, MD: Johns Hopkins University Press.

Dilthey, W. (1887/1996). *Poetry and experience* (Vol. 5). Princeton, NJ: Princeton University Press.

Drinka, T. J., Smith, J. C., & Drinka, P. J. (1987). Correlates of depression and burden for informal caregivers of patients in a geriatrics referral clinic. *Journal of the American Geriatrics Society, 35*(6), 522–525.

Drumond-Andrade, F. C. (2012). Overview. In J. L. Angel, F. Torres-Gil & K. Markides (Eds.), *Aging, health, and longevity in the Mexican-origin population* (pp. 185–192). New York, NY: Springer.

Duncan, W. L. (2012). *The culture of mental health in a changing Oaxaca* (Unpublished doctoral dissertation). University of California, San Diego.

Duncan, W. L. (2017a). Dinámicas ocultas: Culture and psy-sociality in Mexican family constellations therapy. *Ethos, 45*(4), 489–513.

Duncan, W. L. (2017b). Psicoeducación in the land of magical thoughts: Culture and mental-health practice in a changing Oaxaca. *American Ethnologist, 44*(1), 36–51.

Duncan, W. L. (2018). *Transforming therapy: Mental health practice and cultural change in Mexico.* Nashville, TN: Vanderbilt University Press.

Durkheim, E. (1933/1997). *The division of labour in society* (W. Halls, Trans.) New York, NY: Free Press.

Ell, K., & Castañeda, I. (1998). Health care seeking behavior. In S. Loue (Ed.), *Handbook of immigrant health* (pp. 125–143). Boston, MA: Springer.

Esposito, N. (2001). From meaning to meaning: The influence of translation techniques on non-English focus group research. *Qualitative Health Research, 11*(4), 568–579.

Estes, C. (1979). *The aging enterprise: A critical examination of social policies and services for the aged.* Hoboken, NJ: Jossey-Bass.

Estes, C. (2001). *Social policy and aging: A critical perspective.* Thousand Oaks, CA: Sage.

Estes, C., & Binney, E. A. (1989). The biomedicalization of aging: Dangers and dilemmas. *Gerontologist, 29*(5), 587–596.

Fabian, J. (2014). *Time and the other: How anthropology makes its object.* New York, NY: Columbia University Press.

Fairclough, N. (2013). *Critical discourse analysis: The critical study of language* (2nd ed.). Harlow, UK: Pearson.

Fassin, D. (2012). *Humanitarian reason: A moral history of the present.* Berkeley, CA: Univeristy of California Press.

Fine, M. (2017). *Just research in contentious times: Widening the methodological imagination.* New York, NY: Teachers College Press.

Finkler, K. (1997). Gender, domestic violence and sickness in Mexico. *Social Science & Medicine, 45*(8), 1147–1160.

Finkler, K. (2001a). Mistress of lo espiritual. In B. R. Huber & A. R. Sandstrom (Eds.), *Mesoamerican healers* (pp. 117–138). Austin, TX: University of Texas Press.

Finkler, K. (2001b). *Physicians at work, patients in pain: Biomedical practice and patient response in Mexico* (2nd ed.). Durham, NC: Carolina Academic Press.

Fitzsimmons, C. I. (1972). *Susto: An epidemiological study of stress adaptation* (Unpublished doctoral dissertation). University of Texas, Austin.

Foucault, M. (1975). *The birth of the clinic* (A. Sheridan, Trans.) London: Tavistock.

Foucault, M. (1984). The politics of health in the eighteenth century. In P. Rabinow & N. S. Rose (Eds.), *The Foucault Reader* (pp. 273–288.). New York, NY: Pantheon.

Fox, J., & Rivera-Salgado, G. (2004). Building civil society among indigenous migrants. In J. R.-S. Fox, Gaspar (Ed.), *Indigenous Mexican migrants in the United States* (pp. 1–65).

La Jolla, California: Center for U.S.-Mexican Studies and Center for Comparative Immigration Studies.

Fox, P. (1989). From senility to Alzheimer's disease: The rise of the Alzheimer's disease movement. *Milbank Quarterly, 67*(1), 58–102.

Franzen, J. (2007). My father's brain. *How to be alone: Essays.* New York, NY: Macmillan.

Freed, A. O. (1988). Interviewing through an interpreter. *Social Work, 33*(4), 315–319.

Gagnier de Mendoza, M. J. (2005). *Oaxaca celebration: Family, food, and fiestas in Teotitlán.* Santa Fe, NM: Museum of New Mexico Press.

Gaines, A. D. (1987). Alzheimer's disease in the context of black (southern) culture. *Health Matrix, 6*(4), 33–38.

Gaines, A. D. (1992). Ethnopsychiatry: The cultural construction of psychiatries. In A. Gaines (Ed.), *Ethnopsychiatry: The cultural construction of professional and folk psychiatries* (pp. 3–49). Albany, NY: SUNY Press.

Garcia, A. (2010). *The pastoral clinic: Addiction and dispossession along the Rio Grande.* Berkeley, CA: University of California Press.

Gaugler, J. E., Kane, R. L., Kane, R. A., & Newcomer, R. (2006). Predictors of institutionalization in Latinos with dementia. *Journal of Cross-Cultural Gerontology, 21*(3–4), 139–155.

Geertz, C. (1973). *The interpretation of cultures: Selected essays.* New York, NY: Basic Books.

Gelman, C. R. (2012). Familismo and its impact on the family caregiving of Latinos with Alzheimer's disease: A complex narrative. *Research on Aging, 36*(1), 40–71.

Gergen, K. (2009). *An invitation to social construction.* Thousand Oaks, CA: Sage.

Gibbon, S., & Novas, C. (2008). *Genetics, biosociality and the social sciences: Making biologies and identities.* New York, NY: Routledge.

Giddens, A. (2002). *Runaway world.* New York, NY: Routledge.

Giorgi, A. (1985). *Phenomenology and psychological research.* Pittsburgh, PA: Duquesne University Press.

Glass, D. J., & Arnold, S. E. (2012). Some evolutionary perspectives on Alzheimer's disease pathogenesis and pathology. *Alzheimer's & Dementia, 8*(4), 343–351.

Glenn, E. N. (2010). *Forced to care: Coercion and caregiving in America.* Cambridge, MA: Harvard University Press.

Gluckman, M. (1963). Papers in honor of Melville J. Herskovits: Gossip and scandal. *Current Anthropology, 4*(3), 307–316.

Goffman, E. (1961). *Essays on the social situation of mental patients and other inmates.* Garden City, NY: Anchor Books.

Good, B. (1992). Culture and psychopathology: Directions for psychiatric anthropology. In T. Schwartz, G. White, & C. Lutz (Eds.), *New directions in psychological anthropology* (pp. 181–205). Cambridge, UK: Cambridge University Press.

Good, B. (1994). *Medicine, rationality and experience: An anthropological perspective.* Cambridge, UK: Cambridge University Press.

Good, B. (2010). The complexities of psychopharmaceutical hegemonies in Indonesia. In J. H. Jenkins (Ed.), *Pharmaceutical self: The global shaping of experience in an age of psychopharmacology* (pp. 117–144). Santa Fe, NM: SAR Press.

Goodwin, C. (1994). Professional vision. *American Anthropologist, 96*(3), 606–633.

Goody, J. (1976). *Production and reproduction: A comparative study of the domestic domain.* Cambridge. UK: Cambridge University Press.

Grabman, R. (2009). *Gods, gachupines and gringos: A people's history of Mexico.* Mazatlán, Mexico: Editorial Mazatlán.

Graburn, N. H. (2000). What is tradition? *Museum Anthropology, 24*(2–3), 6–11.

Gramsci, A. (1988). *An Antonio Gramsci reader: Selected writings, 1916–1935* (D. Forgacs, Ed.). New York, NY: Schocken Books.

Greenfield, P. M. (2000). What psychology can do for anthropology, or why anthropology took postmodernism on the chin. *American Anthropologist, 102*(3), 564–576.

Guardino, P. (2005). *The time of liberty: Popular political culture in Oaxaca, 1750–1850.* Durham, NC: Duke University Press.

Guarnaccia, P. J. (1997). Social stress and psychological distress among Latinos in the United States. In I. Al-Issa & M. Tousignant (Eds.), *Ethnicity, immigration, and psychopathology* (pp. 71–94). New York, NY: Plenum Press.

Guarnaccia, P. J. (1998). Multicultural experiences of family caregiving: A study of African American, European American, and Hispanic American families. In H. Lefley (Ed.), *Families coping with mental illness: The cultural context* (pp. 45–61). San Francisco, CA: Jossey-Bass.

Guarnaccia, P. J., Lewis-Fernández, R., & Marano, M. R. (2003). Toward a Puerto Rican popular nosology: nervios and ataque de nervios. *Culture, Medicine, and Psychiatry, 27*(3), 339–366.

Guarnaccia, P. J., Good, B. J., & Kleinman, A. (1990). A critical review of epidemiological studies of Puerto Rican mental health. *American Journal of Psychiatry, 147*(11), 1449.

Guarnaccia, P. J., Parka, P., Deschamps, A., Milstein, G., & Argiles, N. (1992). Si dios quiere: Hispanic families' experiences of caring for a seriously mentally-ill family member. *Culture, Medicine, and Psychiatry, 16*(2), 187–215.

Gubrium, J. F. (1972). Toward a socio-environmental theory of aging. *The Gerontologist, 12*(1), 281–284.

Gubrium, J. F., & Holstein, J. A. (2000). *Aging and everyday life.* Oxford, UK: Blackwell.

Gubrium, J. F., & Lynott, R. J. (1987). Measurement and the interpretation of burden in the Alzheimer's disease experience. *Journal of Aging Studies, 1*(3), 265–285.

Gutiérrez, N. C. (2014). Mexico: Availability and cost of health care—legal aspects (LL File No. 2014–010632). Washington, DC: Law Library of Congress, Global Legal Research Center.

Gutmann, M. C. (2007). *Fixing men: Sex, birth control, and AIDS in Mexico.* Berkeley, CA: University of California Press.

Haber, S. H., Klein, H. S., Maurer, N., & Middlebrook, K. (2008). *Mexico since 1980.* Cambridge, UK: Cambridge University Press.

Habermas, J. (2000). Richard Rorty's pragmatic turn. In R. Brandom (Ed.), *Rorty and his critics* (pp. 37–55). Oxford, UK: Blackwell.

Hacking, I. (1986). Making up people. In T. C. Heller, M. Sosna, & D. Wellbery (Eds.), *Reconstructing individualism: Autonomy, individuality, and the self in Western thought* (pp. 222–236). Stanford, CA: Stanford University Press.

Hacking, I. (1998). *Rewriting the soul: Multiple personality and the sciences of memory.* Princeton, NJ: Princeton University Press.

Hacking, I. (1999). *The social construction of what?* Cambridge, MA: Harvard University Press.

Hale, C. R. (2002). Does multiculturalism menace? Governance, cultural rights and the politics of identity in Guatemala. *Journal of Latin American Studies, 34*(3), 485–524.

Han, C. (2012). *Life in debt: Times of care and violence in Neolibral Chile.* Berekley, CA: University of California Press.

Hargrave, T. D., & Anderson, W. T. (2013). *Finishing well: Aging and reparation in the intergenerational family.* New York, NY: Routledge.

Harrington, B. (2003). The social psychology of access in ethnographic research. *Journal of Contemporary Ethnography, 32*(5), 592–625.

Harris, L. (1975). *The myth and reality of aging in America.* Washington, DC: National Council on the Aging.

Harwood, D. G., Barker, W. W., Cantillon, M., Loewenstein, D. A., Ownby, R., & Duara, R. (1998). Depressive symptomatology in first-degree family caregivers of Alzheimer disease patients: A cross-ethnic comparison. *Alzheimer Disease & Associated Disorders, 12*(4), 340–346.

Haviland, J. B. (1977). *Gossip, reputation, and knowledge in Zinacantan.* Chicago, IL: University of Chicago Press.

Hebert, L. E., Weuve, J., Scherr, P. A., & Evans, D. A. (2013). Alzheimer disease in the United States (2010–2050) estimated using the 2010 census. *Neurology, 80*(19), 1778–1783.

Hellier, R. (2001). *Removing the mask: La danza de los viejitos in post-revolution Mexico, 1920–1940* (Unpublished doctoral dissertation). University of Central England, Birmingham.

Henderson, J. N., & Guitierrez-Mayka, M. (1992). Ethnocultural themes in caregiving to Alzheimer's disease patients in Hispanic families. *Clinical Gerontologist, 11*(3–4), 59–74.

Henderson, J. N., & Henderson, L. C. (2002). Cultural construction of disease: A "supernormal" construct of dementia in an American Indian tribe. *Journal of Cross-Cultural Gerontology, 17*(3), 197–212.

Henderson, J. N., & Traphagan, J. W. (2005). Cultural factors in dementia: Perspectives from the anthropology of aging. *Alzheimer Disease & Associated Disorders, 19*(4), 272–274.

Hernández Sáenz, L. M., & Foster, G. M. (2001). Curers and their cures in colonial New Spain and Guatemala: The Spanish component. In B. R. Huber & A. R. Sandstrom (Eds.), *Mesoamerican healers* (pp. 19–46). Austin, TX: University of Texas Press.

Hernández-Díaz, J. & Zafra, G. (2007). *Artesanos y artesanas: Creacion, innovacion y tradicion en la produccion de artesanias.* Madrid, Spain: Plaza y Valdes.

Hernández-Díaz, J. (2012). *La danza de la pluma en Teotitlán del Valle: Expresión de identidad de una comunidad Zapoteca.* Oaxaca, Mexico: Collección Diálogos.

Herrera, A. P., Angel, J. L., Venegas, C. D., & Angel, R. J. (2012). Estimating the demand for long-term care among aging Mexican Americans: Cultural preferences versus economic realities. In J. L. Angel, F. Torres-Gil, & K. Markides (Eds.), *Aging, health, and longevity in the Mexican-origin population* (pp. 259–276). New York, NY: Springer.

Higgins, C. M. (1975). Integrative aspects of folk and western medicine among the urban poor of Oaxaca. *Anthropological Quarterly, 48*(1), 31–37.

Hinton, D. E., Hinton, A. L., Eng, K. T., & Choung, S. (2012). PTSD and key somatic complaints and cultural syndromes among rural Cambodians: The results of a needs assessment survey. *Medical Anthropology Quarterly, 26*(3), 383–407.

Hinton, D. E., & Lewis-Fernández, R. (2010). Idioms of distress among trauma survivors: subtypes and clinical utility. *Culture, Medicine, and Psychiatry, 34*(2), 209–218.

Hinton, D. E., Pich, V., Marques, L., Nickerson, A., & Pollack, M. H. (2010). Khyâl attacks: A key idiom of distress among traumatized Cambodia refugees. *Culture, Medicine, and Psychiatry, 34*(2), 244–78.

Hinton, L., Franz, C., & Friend, J. (2004). Pathways to dementia diagnosis: Evidence for cross-ethnic differences. *Alzheimer Disease & Associated Disorders, 18*(3), 134–144.

Hobsbawm, E., & Ranger, T. (1983) *The invention of tradition.* Cambridge, UK: Cambridge University Press.

Hollan, D. (2008). Being there: On the imaginative aspects of understanding others and being understood. *Ethos, 36*(4), 475–489.

Hollan, D., & Throop, C. J. (2008). Whatever happened to empathy?: Introduction. *Ethos, 36*(4), 385–401.

Holmes, S. (2013). *Fresh fruit, broken bodies: Migrant farmworkers in the United States.* Berkeley, CA: University of California Press.

Holstein, J. A., & Gubrium, J. F. (2012). *The self we live by: Narrative identity in a postmodern world.* Oxford, UK: Oxford University Press.

Holstein, M. B., & Minkler, M. (2007). Critical gerontology: Reflections for the 21st Century. In T. Scharf & M. Bernard (Eds.), *Critical perspectives on ageing societies* (pp. 13–26). Bristol, UK: Policy Press.

Hook, J. N., Davis, D. E., Owen, J., Worthington Jr., E. L., & Utsey, S. O. (2013). Cultural humility: Measuring openness to culturally diverse clients. *Journal of Counseling Psychology, 60*(3), 353.

Horner, A. E. (1990). The *assumption of tradition: Creating, collecting, and conserving cultural artifacts in the Cameroon grassfields (West Africa)* (Unpublished doctoral dissertation). University of California, Berkeley.

Hunt, L. L. M. (1992). *Living with cancer in Oaxaca, Mexico: Patient and physician perspectives in cultural context* (Unpublished doctoral dissertation). Harvard University, Cambridge, MA.

Husserl, E., (1913/1963). *Ideas: A general introduction to pure phenomenology.* (W. R. B. Gibson, Trans.) New York, NY: Collier Books.

Husserl, E. (1900/1970). *Logical investigations* (Vol. 1, J. Findlay, Trans.). New York, NY: Routledge.

INEGI. (2014). *An approach to Mexico* (4th ed.). Aguascalientes, Mexico: Aguascalientes Instituto Nacional de Estadística y Geografía.

Jackson, M. (2017). *How lifeworlds work: Emotionality, sociality, and the ambiguity of being.* Chicago, IL: University of Chicago Press.

Jackson, R. (2005). Building human capital in an aging Mexico: A Report of the U.S.-Mexico Binational Council. Washington, DC: Center for Strategic and International Studies.

Jakobsen, H. (2012). Focus groups and methodological rigour outside the minority world: Making the method work to its strengths in Tanzania. *Qualitative Research, 12*(2), 111–130.

James, W. (1907/2000). *Pragmatism and other writings.* New York, NY: Penguin.

Jervis, L. L. (2001). The pollution of incontinence and the dirty work of caregiving in a US nursing home. *Medical Anthropology Quarterly, 15*(1), 84–99.

Jiménez, C. (2014, August 25). Abandono y maltrado, la realidad. *Síntesis,* pp. 4–5.

Jodelet, D. (1991). *Madness and social representations: Living with the mad in one French community* (T. Pownall, Trans. & G. Duveen, Ed.). Berkeley, CA: University of California Press.

Kaiser, B. N., Kohrt, B. A., Keys, H. M., Khoury, N. M., & Brewster, A. R. T. (2013). Strategies for assessing mental health in Haiti: Local instrument development and transcultural translation. *Transcultural Psychiatry, 50*(4), 532–558.

Kearney, M. (1995). The effects of transnational culture, economy, and migration on Mixtec identity in Oaxacalifornia. In M. P. Smith & J. R. Feagin (Eds.), *The bubbling cauldron: Race, ethnicity, and the urban crisis* (pp. 226–243). Minneapolis, MN: University of Minnesota Press.

Keefe, S., Padilla, A., & Carlos, M. (1979). The Mexican-American extended family as an emotional support system. *Human Organization, 38*(2), 144–152.

Keller, R. (2011). The Sociology of Knowledge Approach to Discourse (SKAD). *Human Studies, 34*(1), 43–65.

Kendall, G., & Wickham, G. (1998). *Using Foucault's methods.* Thousand Oaks, CA: Sage.

Kidd, P. S., & Parshall, M. B. (2000). Getting the focus and the group: Enhancing analytical rigor in focus group research. *Qualitative health research, 10*(3), 293–308.

Kirmayer, L. (1994). Improvisation and authority in illness meaning. *Culture, Medicine, and Psychiatry, 18*(2), 183–214.

Kirmayer, L. (2012). Rethinking cultural competence. *Transcultural Psychiatry*, 49(2), 149–164.

Kitwood, T. (1997). *Dementia reconsidered: The person comes first.* Buckingham, UK: Open University Press.

Kleinman, A. (1980). *Patients and healers in the context of culture: An exploration of the borderland between anthropology, medicine, and psychiatry.* Berkeley, CA: University of California Press.

Kleinman, A. (1988a). *The illness narratives: Suffering, healing, and the human condition.* New York, NY: Basic Books.

Kleinman, A. (1988b). *Rethinking psychiatry: From cultural category to personal experience.* New York, NY: Free Press.

Kleinman, A. (1997). *Writing at the margin: Discourse between anthropology and medicine.* Berkeley, CA: University of California Press.

Kleinman, A. (2008). Catastrophe and caregiving: The failure of medicine as an art. *The Lancet*, 371(9606), 22–23.

Kleinman, A. (2009). Caregiving: The odyssey of becoming more human. *The Lancet*, 373(9660), 292–93.

Kleinman, A. (2010). Four social theories for global health. *The Lancet*, 375(9725), 1518–1519.

Kleinman, A., Das, V., & Lock, M. M. (1997). *Social suffering.* Berkeley, CA: University of California Press.

Kleinman, A., & Fitz-Henry, E. (2007). The experiential basis of subjectivity: How individuals change in the context of societal transformation. In Biehl, J., Good, B., & Kleinman, A. (Eds.) *Subjectivity: Ethnographic investigations* (pp. 52–65). Berkeley, CA: University of California Press.

Kleinman, A., & Hanna, B. (2008). Catastrophe, caregiving and today's biomedicine. *BioSocieties*, 3(3), 287–301.

Knight, A. (1990). Racism, revolution, and indigenismo: Mexico, 1910–1940. In R. Graham (Ed.), *The idea of race in Latin America, 1870–1940* (pp. 71–113). Austin, TX: University of Texas Press.

Kohrt, B. A., Rasmussen, A., Kaiser, B. N., Haroz, E. E., Maharjan, S. M., Mutamba, B. B., . . . & Hinton, D. E. (2013). Cultural concepts of distress and psychiatric disorders: Literature review and research recommendations for global mental health epidemiology. *International Journal of Epidemiology*, 43(2), 365–406.

Krueger, R. A. (2009). *Focus groups: A practical guide for applied research.* Thousand Oaks, CA: Sage.

Kunow, R. (2010). Old age and globalization. In T. Cole, R. Ray, & R. Kastenbaum (Eds.), *A guide to humanistic studies in aging: What does it mean to grow old* (pp. 293–318). Baltimore, MD: Johns Hopkins University Press.

Lakoff, G., & Johnson, M. (1980). *Metaphors we live by.* Chicago, IL: University of Chicago Press.

Larkey, L. K., Hecht, M. L., Miller, K., & Alatorre, C. (2001). Hispanic cultural norms for health-seeking behaviors in the face of symptoms. *Health Education & Behavior, 28*(1), 65–80.

Latour, B. (2004). Why has critique run out of steam? From matters of fact to matters of concern. *Critical Inquiry, 30*(2), 225–248.

Latour, B. (1993). *We have never been modern.* Cambridge, MA: Harvard University Press.

Latour, B. (2007). *Reassembling the social.* Oxford, UK: Oxford University Press.

Laubscher, L. (2016). Introduction to psychology as a human science. San Diego, CA: Cognella.

Laugier, S. (2013). *Why we need ordinary language philosophy.* Chicago, IL: University of Chicago Press.

Leibing, A. (2002). Flexible hips? On Alzheimer's disease and aging in Brazil. *Journal of Cross-Cultural Gerontology, 17*(3), 213–232.

Leinaweaver, J. B. (2010). Outsourcing care: How Peruvian migrants meet transnational family obligations. *Latin American Perspectives, 37*(5), 67–87.

León-Portilla, M. (2012). *Aztec thought and culture: A study of the ancient Nahuatl mind.* Norman, OK: University of Oklahoma Press.

Leslie, C. (1980). Medical pluralism in world perspective. *Social Science & Medicine. Part B: Medical Anthropology, 14*(4), 191–195.

Levinas, E. (1992). *Totality and infinity: An essay on exteriority* (A. Lingis, Trans.). Pittsburgh, PA: Duquesne University Press.

Levinas, E. (1998a). *Entre nous: On thinking-of-the-other* (M. Smith & B. Harshav, Trans.). New York, NY: Columbia University Press.

Levinas, E. (1998b). *Otherwise than being: Or beyond essence* (A. Lingis, Trans.). Pittsburgh, PA: Duquesne University Press.

Lewis, S. E. (2006). The nation, education, and the "Indian problem" in Mexico, 1920–1940. In M. K. L. Vaughan & S. Lewis (Eds.), *The eagle and the virgin: Nation and cultural revolution in Mexico, 1920–1940* (pp. 176–195). Durham, NC: Duke University Press.

Lewis-Fernández, R., Gorritz, M., Raggio, G. A., Peláez, C., Chen, H., & Guarnaccia, P. J. (2010). Association of trauma-related disorders and dissociation with four idioms of distress among Latino psychiatric outpatients. *Culture, Medicine, and Psychiatry, 34*(2), 219–243.

Lin, K.-M., Inui, T. S., Kleinman, A. M., & Womack, W. M. (1982). Sociocultural determinants of the help-seeking behavior of patients with mental illness. *Journal of Nervous and Mental Disease, 170*(2), 78–85.

Lind, M. (2015). *Ancient Zapotec religion: An ethnohistorical and archaeological perspective.* Denver, CO: University Press of Colorado.

Lock, M. (1997). Displaced suffering: The reconstruction of death in North America and Japan. In A. Kleinman, V. Das, & M. M. Lock (Eds.), *Social suffering* (pp. 207–244). Berkeley, CA: University of California Press.

Lock, M. (2007). Biosociality and susceptibility genes: A cautionary tale. In S. Gibbon & C. Novas (Eds.), *Biosocialities, genetics and the social sciences: Making biologies and identities* (pp. 56–78). New York, NY: Routledge.

Lock, M. (2013). *The Alzheimer conundrum: Entanglements of dementia and aging.* Princeton, NJ: Princeton University Press.

Lock, M., & Nichter, M. (2002). From documenting medical pluralism to critical interpretations of globalized health knowledge, policies, and practices. In M. Lock & M. Nichter (Eds.), *New horizons in medical anthropology: Essays in honour of Charles Leslie* (pp. 1–35). New York, NY: Routledge.

Lyons, H. Z., Johnson, A., Bike, D. H., Flores, L. Y., Ojeda, L., & Rosales, R. (2013). Qualitative research as social justice practice with culturally diverse populations. *Journal for Social Action in Counseling and Psychology, 5*(2), 10–25

MacCannell, D. (1984). Reconstructed ethnicity tourism and cultural identity in third world communities. *Annals of Tourism Research, 11*(3), 375–391.

Mace, N. L., & Rabins, P. V. (2011). *The 36-hour day: A family guide to caring for people who have Alzheimer disease, related dementias, and memory loss* (5th ed.). Baltimore, MD: Johns Hopkins University Press.

Madriz, E. I. (1998). Using focus groups with lower socioeconomic status Latina women. *Qualitative Inquiry, 4*(1), 114–128.

Mahoney, R., Regan, C., Katona, C., & Livingston, G. (2005). Anxiety and depression in family caregivers of people with Alzheimer disease: The LASER–A.D. study. *American Journal of Geriatric Psychiatry, 13*(9), 795–801.

Marcus, G. E. (1995). Ethnography in/of the world system: The emergence of multi-sited ethnography. *Annual Review of Anthropology, 24,* 95–117.

Marcus, J., & Flannery, K. V. (1996). *Zapotec civilization: How urban society evolved in Mexico's Oaxaca valley.* London, UK: Thames and Hudson.

Marcus, J., & Flannery, K. V. (2000). Cultural evolution in Oaxaca: The origins of the Zapotec and Mixtec civilizations. In R. E. W. Adams & M. J. MacLeod (Eds.), *The Cambridge history of the native peoples of the Americas, Part 1* (Vol. 2, pp. 358–406). Cambridge, UK: Cambridge University Press.

Margulies, D. S. (2012). The salmon of doubt. In S. S. Choudhury & J. Slaby (Eds.), *Critical neuroscience: A handbook of the social and cultural contexts of neuroscience* (pp. 273–285). New York, NY: Blackwell.

Martinez Tyson, D. D., Castaneda, H., Porter, M., Quiroz, M., & Carrion, I. (2011). More similar than different? Exploring cultural models of depression among Latino immigrants in Florida. *Depression Research and Treatment, 11*(1), 1–11.

Matthew, L., Matthew, L. E., & Oudijk, M. (Eds.). (2007). *Indian conquistadors: Indigenous allies in the conquest of Mesoamerica.* Norman, OK: University of Oklahoma Press.

McDowell, J. (2000). Towards rehabilitating objectivity. In R. Brandom (Ed.), *Rory and his critics* (pp. 109–123). Oxford, UK: Blackwell.

McMullen, L. (2011). A discursive analysis of Teresa's protocol: Enhancing oneself, diminishing others. In F. Wertz, K. Charmaz, L. McMullen, R. Josselson, R. Anderson, & E. McSpadden (Eds.), *Five ways of doing qualitative analysis: Phenomenological psychology, grounded theory, discourse analysis, narrative research, and intuitive inquiry* (pp. 205–233). New York, NY: Guilford Press.

McWilliams, N. (2011). *Psychoanalytic diagnosis: Understanding personality structure in the clinical process.* New York, NY: Guilford Press.

Menéndez, E. (1994). La enfermedad y la curación ¿Qué es medicina tradicional? *Alteridades, 4*(7), 71–83.

Merleau-Ponty, M. (1945/1962). *Phenomenology of perception* (C. Smith, Trans.). New York, NY: Routledge.

Merry, S. E. (2009). *Human rights and gender violence: Translating international law into local justice.* Chicago, IL: University of Chicago Press.

Merton, R. K., Lowenthal, M. F., & Kendall, P. L. (1990). *The focussed interview: A manual.* Florence, MA: Free Press.

Metzl, J. M., & Hansen, H. (2014). Structural competency: Theorizing a new medical engagement with stigma and inequality. *Social Science & Medicine, 103,* 126–133.

Mies, M. (1983). *Towards a methodology for feminist research.* In G. Bowles & D. Klein (Eds.) (pp. 139–152). Theories of Women's Studies. London, UK: Routledge.

Miller, D. A. (1981). The "sandwich" generation: Adult children of the aging. *Social Work, 26*(5), 419–423.

Mol, A. (2008). *The logic of care: Health and the problem of patient choice.* New York, NY: Routledge.

Mol, A., Moser, I., & Pols, J. (2010). *Care in practice: On tinkering in clinics, homes and farms.* New Brunswick, NJ: Transaction Publishers.

Monin, J. K., & Schulz, R. (2009). Interpersonal effects of suffering in older adult caregiving relationships. *Psychology and Aging, 24*(3), 681.

Morales, R. G. R., & Cruz, A. S. G. (2002). Características de la migración internacional en las regiones mixteca y valles Centrales del estado de Oaxaca. https://www.colef.mx/sepmig/wp-content/uploads/2013/05/8va-Rafael-Reyes-La-migraci%C3%B3n-oaxaque%C3%B1a.pdf.

Morris, C. W. (1971). *Writings on the general theory of signs.* The Hague, Netherlands: Mouton Press.

Moscovici, S. (2000). *Social representations: Explorations in social psychology* (G. Duveen, Ed.). Cambridge, MA: Polity Press.

Moscovici, S. (2008). *Psychoanalysis: Its image and its public* (D. Macey, Trans., & G. Duveen, Ed.). Malden, MA: Polity Press.

Mourao, R. J., Mansur, G., Malloy-Diniz, L. F., Castro Costa, E., & Diniz, B. S. (2016). Depressive symptoms increase the risk of progression to dementia in subjects with mild cognitive impairment: Systematic review and meta-analysis. *International Journal of Geriatric Psychiatry, 31*(8), 905–911.

Murphy, A. D., & Stepick, A. (1991). *Social inequality in Oaxaca: A history of resistance and change.* Philadelphia, PA: Temple University Press.

Myers, G. (1998). Displaying opinions: Topics and disagreement in focus groups. *Language in Society, 27*(1), 85–111.

Napolitano, V. (2002). *Migration, mujercitas, and medicine men: Living in urban Mexico.* Berkeley, CA: University of California Press.

Nell, V. (1999). Luria in Uzbekistan: The vicissitudes of cross-cultural neuropsychology. *Neuropsychology Review, 9*(1), 45–52.

Nichter, M. (1978). Part Two: Patterns of resort in the use of therapy systems and their significance for health planning in South Asia. *Medical Anthropology, 2*(2), 29–56.

Nichter, M. (1981). Idioms of distress: Alternatives in the expression of psychosocial distress: A case study from South India. *Culture, Medicine, and Psychiatry, 5*(4), 379–408.

Nichter, M. (2008). *Global health: Why cultural perceptions, social representations, and biopolitics matter.* Tucson, AZ: University of Arizona Press.

Nichter, M. (2010). Idioms of distress revisited. *Culture, Medicine, and Psychiatry, 34*(2), 401–416.

Norget, K. (2006). *Days of death, days of life: Ritual in the popular culture of Oaxaca.* New York, NY: Columbia University Press.

Norris, J. E., Pratt, M. W., & Kuiack, S. L. (2003). Parent-child relations in adulthood: An intergenerational family systems perspective. In L. Kuczynski (Ed.), *Handbook of dynamics in parent-child relations* (pp. 325–344). Thousand Oaks, CA: Sage.

Nuckolls, C. W. (1991). Deciding how to decide: Possession-mediumship in Jalari divination. *Medical Anthropology, 13*(1–2), 57–82.

Obeyesekere, G. (1990). *The work of culture: Symbolic transformation in psychoanalysis and anthropology.* Chicago, IL: University of Chicago Press.

Ochs, E., & Kremer-Sadlik, T. (2015). How postindustrial families talk. *Annual Review of Anthropology, 44*, 87–103.

OECD. (2015). OECD better life index. http://www.oecdbetterlifeindex.org/countries /mexico/.

Ordóñez, M. d. J. (2000). El territorio del estado de Oaxaca: Una revisión histórica. *Investigaciones geográficas,* (42), 67–86.

Ortiz, F. A., Davis, K. G., & McNeill, B. W. (2008). Curanderismo: Religious and spiritual worldviews and indigenous healing traditions. In B. McNeil & J. Cervantes (Eds.), *Latina/o healing practices: Mestizo and indigenous perspectives* (pp. 271–300). New York, NY: Routledge.

Oudijk, M. (2000). *Historiography of the Bènizàa: The postclassic and early colonial periods (1000–1600 A.D.).* Leiden, Netherlands: Universiteit Leiden.

Ownby, R. L., Crocco, E., Acevedo, A., John, V., & Loewenstein, D. (2006). Depression and risk for Alzheimer disease: Systematic review, meta-analysis, and metaregression analysis. *Archives of General Psychiatry, 63*(5), 530–538.

Packer, M. (2010a). Educational research as a reflexive science of constitution. *Yearbook of the National Society for the Study of Education, 109*(1), 17–33.

Packer, M. (2010b). *The science of qualitative research.* Cambridge, UK: Cambridge University Press.

Padilla, A. M., & De Snyder, V. N. S. (1988). Psychology in pre-Columbian Mexico. *Hispanic Journal of Behavioral Sciences, 10*(1), 55–66.

Papps, E., & Ramsden, I. (1996). Cultural safety in nursing: The New Zealand experience. *International Journal of Quality in Health Care, 8*(5), 491–497.

Parker, I. (1998). *Social constructionism, discourse and realism.* Thousand Oaks, CA: Sage.

Parreñas, R. S. (2005). *Children of global migration: Transnational families and gendered woes.* Stanford, CA: Stanford University Press.

Parreñas, R. (2015). *Servants of globalization: Migration and domestic work.* Stanford, CA: Stanford University Press.

Partida-Bush, V. (2005, August/September). Demographic transition, demographic bonus and ageing in Mexico. *Proceedings of the United Nations Expert Group Meeting on Social and Economic Implications of Changing Population Age Structures,* Mexico City, Mexico, 285–307.

Pierce, C. S. (1905). What pragmatism is. *The Monist, 15*(2), 161–181.

Pigg, S. L. (1995). The social symbolism of healing in Nepal. *Ethnology, 34*(1), 17–36.

Pigg, S. L. (1996). The credible and the credulous: The question of "villagers' beliefs" in Nepal. *Cultural Anthropology, 11*(2), 160–201.

Post, S. G. (2000). *The moral challenge of Alzheimer disease: Ethical issues from diagnosis to dying* (2nd ed.). Baltimore, MD: Johns Hopkins University Press.

Potter, J. (2003). Discourse analysis and discursive psychology. In D. Fox & I. Prillentesky (Eds.), *Qualitative research in psychology: Expanding perspectives in methodology and design* (pp. 73–94). Washington, DC: American Psychological Association.

Potter, J., & Wetherell, M. (1987). *Discourse and social psychology: Beyond attitudes and behaviour.* Thousand Oaks, CA: Sage.

Pouillon, J. (2016). Remarks on the verb "to believe." *Journal of Ethnographic Theory, 6*(3), 485–492.

Prince, M., Wimo, A., Guerchet, M., Ali G,-C., Wu, T.-Z., & Prina, M., (2015). *World Alzheimer report 2015: The global impact of dementia: An analysis of prevalence, incidence, cost and trends.* London: Alzheimer's Disease International.

Rabinow, P. (1996). Artificiality and enlightenment: From sociobiology to biosociality. *Essays on the anthropology of reason* (pp. 91–111). Princeton, NJ: Princeton University Press.

Ramírez Stege, A. M., & Yarris, K. E. (2017). Culture in la clínica: Evaluating the utility of the Cultural Formulation Interview (CFI) in a Mexican outpatient setting. *Transcultural Psychiatry, 54*(4), 466–487.

Rautman, A. L. (1962). Role reversal in geriatrics. *Mental Hygiene, 46,* 116–120.

Redfield, R. (1941). *The folk culture of Yucatan.* Chicago, IL: University of Chicago Press.

Religion & Ethics NewsWeekly. (2011, July 25). *Arthur Kleinman on caregiving* [Video file]. http://www.youtube.com/watch?v=UxosTKujwWQ.

Riessman, C. K. (2002). Doing justice: Positioning the interpreter in narrative work. In Wendy Patterson (Ed.), *Strategic narrative: New perspectives on the power of personal and cultural stories* (pp. 195–216). Lanham, MA: Lexington Books.

Robbins, J. (2013). Beyond the suffering subject: Toward an anthropology of the good. *Journal of the Royal Anthropological Institute, 19*(3), 447–462.

Robinson Shurgot, G. S., & Knight, B. G. (2005). Preliminary study investigating acculturation, cultural values, and psychological distress in Latino caregivers of dementia patients. *Hispanic Health Care International, 3*(1), 37–44.

Romanyshyn, R. D. (2012). The necessity for the humanities in psychology: The psychologist and his/her shadow. *Humanistic Psychologist, 40*(3), 234–245.

Rorty, R. (1979). *Philosophy and the mirror of nature.* Princeton, NJ: Princeton University Press.

Rorty, R. (1982). *Consequences of pragmatism: Essays, 1972–1980.* Minneapolis, MN: University of Minnesota Press.

Rose, N. (1998). *Inventing our selves: Psychology, power, and personhood.* Cambridge, UK: Cambridge University Press.

Rose, N. (2007). *The politics of life itself: Biomedicine, power, and subjectivity in the twenty-first century.* Princeton, NJ: Princeton University Press.

Rowe, J. W., & Kahn, R. L. (1987). Human aging: Usual and successful. *Science, 237*(4811), 143–149.

Rowe, J. W., & Kahn, R. L. (1997). Successful aging. *Gerontologist, 37*(4), 433–440.

Royce, A. P. (2011). *Becoming an ancestor: The Isthmus Zapotec way of death.* Albany, NY: SUNY Press.

Rubel, A. J. (1960). Concepts of disease in Mexican-American culture. *American Anthropologist, 62*(5), 795–814.

Rubel, A. J., & Browner, C. (1999). Antropología de la salud en Oaxaca. *Alteridades, 9*(17).

Ruiz Balzola, A. (2014). Construyendo Teotitlán: Tapetes, migrantes, gringos y etnógrafos. *Aibr-Revista De Antropologia Iberoamericana, 9*(1), 53–73.

Ryan, J., Al Sheedi, Y. M., White, G., & Watkins, D. (2015). Respecting the culture: undertaking focus groups in Oman. *Qualitative Research, 15*(3), 373–388.

Sabat, S. R., & Harré, R. (1992). The construction and deconstruction of self in Alzheimer's disease. *Ageing and Society, 12*(4), 443–461.

Sacks, O. (1998). *The man who mistook his wife for a hat: And other clinical tales.* New York, NY: Simon and Schuster.

Sacks, O. (2012). *Oaxaca journal.* New York, NY: Random House.

Said, E. (1978). *Orientalism.* New York, NY: Vintage.

Saldaña, J. (2012). *The coding manual for qualitative researchers.* Thousand Oaks, CA: Sage Publications.

Sault, N. L. (1985). *Zapotec godmothers: The centrality of women for "compadrazgo" groups in a village of Oaxaca, Mexico* (Unpublished doctoral dissertation). University of California, Los Angeles.

Scheper-Hughes, N. (1993). *Death without weeping: The violence of everyday life in Brazil*. Berkeley, CA: University of California Press.

Schulz, R. (2000). *Handbook on dementia caregiving: Evidence-based interventions for family caregivers* (R. Schulz, Ed.). New York, NY: Springer.

Schulz, R., & Williamson, G. M. (1991). A 2-year longitudinal study of depression among Alzheimer's caregivers. *Psychology and Aging*, *6*(4), 569.

Scott, M. A. (2012). Paying down the care deficit: The health consequences for grand-mothers caring for grandchildren in a Mexican migrant community of origin. *Anthropology & Aging*, 33(4), 142–152.

Secretaría de Salud. (2007). *Programa de acción específico (2007–2012): Medicina tradicional y sistemas complementarios de atención a la salud*. Mexico City, Mexico: Secretaría de Salud.

Secretaría de Salud. (2010) *Programa de acción en salud mental*. Mexico City, Mexico: Secretaría de Salud.

SEDESOL. (2014). *Teotitlán Del Valle, Oaxaca: Informe anual sobre la situación de pobreza y rezago social*. Mexico City, Mexico: SEDESOL.

Seltzer, M. M. (1990). Role reversal: You don't go home again. *Journal of Gerontological Social Work*, *15*(1–2), 5–14.

Selye, H. (1956). *The stress of life*. New York, NY: McGraw-Hill.

Sesia, P. M. (1996). "Women come here on their own when they need to": Prenatal care, authoritative knowledge, and maternal health in Oaxaca. *Medical Anthropology Quarterly*, *10*(2), 121–140.

Sesia, P. M. (2001). Aquí la PROGRESA está muy dura: Estado, negociación e identidad entre familias indígenas rurales. *Desacatos*, (8), 109–128.

Slone, L. B., Norris, F. H., Murphy, A. D., Baker, C. K., Perilla, J. L., Diaz, D., . . . de Jesús Gutiérrez Rodriguez, J. (2006). Epidemiology of major depression in four cities in Mexico. *Depression and Anxiety*, *23*(3), 158–167.

Smith, B. D. (1997). The initial domestication of Cucurbita pepo in the Americas 10,000 years ago. *Science*, *276*(5314), 932–934.

Smith-Morris, C., Morales-Campos, D., Alvarez, E. A. C., & Turner, M. (2013). An anthropology of *familismo*: On narratives and description of Mexican/immigrants. *Hispanic Journal of Behavioral Sciences*, *35*(1), 35–60.

Smith-Oka, V. (2013). *Shaping the motherhood of indigenous Mexico*. Nashville, TN: Vanderbilt University Press.

Snowdon, D. A. (1997). Aging and Alzheimer's disease: Lessons from the Nun Study. *Gerontologist*, *37*(2), 150–156.

Somolinos d'Ardois, G. (1973). *La medicina en las culturas mesoamericanas anteriores a la conquista* (Vol. 1). Mexico City, Mexico: Sociedad Mexicana de Historia y Filosofía de la Medicina.

Somolinos d'Ardois, G. (1976). *Historia de la psiquiatría en México*. Mexico City, Mexico: Secretaría de Educación Pública, Dirección General de Divulgación.

Sontag, S. (2001). *Illness as metaphor and AIDS and its metaphors.* New York, NY: Picador.

Squires, A. (2009). Methodological challenges in cross-language qualitative research: A research review. *International Journal of Nursing Studies, 46*(2), 277–287.

Stahler-Sholk, R. (2007). Resisting neoliberal homogenization: The Zapatista autonomy movement. *Latin American Perspectives, 34*(2), 48–63.

Stephen, L. (2005). *Zapotec women: Gender, class, and ethnicity in globalized Oaxaca* (2nd ed.). Durham, NC: Duke University Press.

Stephen, L. (2007). *Transborder lives: Indigenous Oaxacans in Mexico, California, and Oregon.* Durham, NC: Duke University Press.

Stephen, L. (2013). *We are the face of Oaxaca: Testimony and social movements.* Durham, NC: Duke University Press.

Suchman, L., & Jordan, B. (1990). Interactional troubles in face-to-face survey interviews. *Journal of the American Statistical Association, 85*(409), 232–241.

Sue, S., Fujino, D. C., Hu, L. T., Takeuchi, D. T., & Zane, N. W. (1991). Community mental health services for ethnic minority groups: A test of the cultural responsiveness hypothesis. *Journal of Consulting and Clinical Psychology, 59*(4), 533–540.

Tarlow, B. J., Wisniewski, S. R., Belle, S. H., Rubert, M., Ory, M. G., & Gallagher-Thompson, D. (2004). Positive aspects of caregiving: Contributions of the REACH project to the development of new measures for Alzheimer's caregiving. *Research on Aging, 26*(4), 429–453.

Taylor, W. B. (1979). *Drinking, homicide, and rebellion in colonial Mexican villages.* Stanford, CA: Stanford University Press.

Temple, B. (2002). Crossed wires: Interpreters, translators, and bilingual workers in cross-language research. *Qualitative Health Research, 12*(6), 844–854.

Temple, B., & Edwards, R. (2008). Interpreters/translators and cross-language research: Reflexivity and border crossings. *International Journal of Qualitative Methods, 1*(2), 1–12.

Tervalon, M., & Murray-Garcia, J. (1998). Cultural humility versus cultural competence: A critical distinction in defining physician training outcomes in multicultural education. *Journal of Health Care for the Poor and Underserved, 9*(2), 117–125.

Ticktin, M. I. (2011). *Casualties of care: Immigration and the politics of humanitarianism in France.* Berkeley, CA: University of California Press.

Traphagan, J. W. (1998). Localizing senility: Illness and agency among older Japanese. *Journal of Cross-Cultural Gerontology, 13*(1), 81–98.

Treviño, C. V. (2001). Curanderismo in Mexico and Guatemala: Its historical evolution from the sixteenth to the nineteenth century. In B. R. Huber & A. R. Sandstrom (Eds.), *Mesoamerican healers* (pp. 47–65). Austin, TX: University of Texas Press.

United Nations Department of Economic and Social Affairs. (2002). *Executive summary. World population ageing, 1950–2050.* New York, NY: United Nations.

van den Berg, J. H. (1987). The rise and fall of the medical model in psychiatry. The Silverman Conference, Duquesne University, Pittsburgh, PA.

Van Gameren, E. (2010). Health insurance and use of alternative medicine in Mexico. *Health Policy, 98*(1), 50–57.

van Manen, M. (2004). Lived experience. In M. Lewis-Beck, A. Bryman, & T. Liao (Eds.), *The SAGE encyclopedia of social science research methods* (Vol. 2, pp. 579–580). Thousand Oaks, CA: Sage.

Vargas-Barón, E. (1968). *Development and change of rural artisanry: Weaving industries of the Oaxaca Valley, Mexico* (unpublished doctoral dissertation). Stanford University, Stanford, CA.

Wacquant, L. (2011). Habitus as topic and tool: Reflections on becoming a prizefighter. *Qualitative Research in Psychology, 8*(1), 81–92.

Wadley, V. G., & Haley, W. E. (2001). Diagnostic attributions versus labeling impact of Alzheimer's disease and major depression diagnoses on emotions, beliefs, and helping intentions of family members. *Journals of Gerontology Series B: Psychological Sciences and Social Sciences, 56*(4), 244–252.

Walsh, R. (2003). The methods of reflexivity. *Humanistic Psychologist, 31*(4), 51–66.

Weiner, B. (1993). On sin versus sickness: A theory of perceived responsibility and social motivation. *American Psychologist, 48*(9), 957.

Wentzell, E. (2013). *Maturing masculinities: Aging, chronic illness, and viagra in Mexico.* Durham, NC: Duke University Press.

Wentzell, E. (2015). Medical research participation as citizenship: Modeling modern masculinity and marriage in a Mexican sexual health study. *American Anthropologist, 117*(4), 652–664.

White, M. (2009). *A philosophy of culture: The scope of holistic pragmatism.* Princeton, NJ: Princeton University Press.

Whitecotton, J. W. (1977). *The Zapotecs: Princes, priests, and peasants.* Norman, OK: University of Oklahoma Press.

Whitecotton, J. W. (1992). Culture and exchange in postclassic Oaxaca. In E. Schortman & P. A. Urban (Eds.), *Resources, power, and interregional interaction* (pp. 51–74). New York, NY: Springer.

Whiteford, M. B. (1995). Como se cura: Patterns of medical choice among working class families in the city of Oaxaca, Mexico. In D. M. Warren, L. J. Slikkerveer, D. Brokensha, & W. H. Dechering (Eds.), *The cultural dimension of development* (pp. 218–230). Rugby, UK: Practical Action Publishing.

Whitley, R. (2007). Cultural competence, evidence-based medicine, and evidence-based practices. *Psychiatric Services, 58*(12), 1588–1590.

Wilk, R. (2006). *Home cooking in the global village: Caribbean food from buccaneers to ecotourists.* New York, NY: Bloomsbury Academic.

Wilkinson, I., & Kleinman, A. (2016). *A passion for society: How we think about human suffering.* Berkeley, CA: University of California Press.

Williams, R. (1977). *Marxism and literature* (Vol. 1). Oxford, UK: Oxford University Press.

Wong, R., & Palloni, A. (2009). Aging in Mexico and Latin America. In P. Uhlenberg (Ed.), *International handbook of population aging* (Vol. 2, pp. 231–252). New York, NY: Springer.

Wood, L. A., & Kroger, R. O. (2000). *Doing discourse analysis: Methods for studying action in talk and text*. Thousand Oaks, CA: Sage.

Wood, W. W. (2000). Flexible production, households, and fieldwork: Multisited Zapotec weavers in the era of late capitalism. *Ethnology, 39*(2), 133–148.

Wood, W. W. (2008). *Made in Mexico: Zapotec weavers and the global ethnic art market*. Bloomington, IN: Indiana University Press.

Worthen, H. M. (2012). *The presence of absence: Indigenous migration, a ghost town, and the remaking of gendered communal systems in Oaxaca, Mexico* (Unpublished doctoral dissertation). University of North Carolina, Chapel Hill.

Worthen, H. (2015). Indigenous women's political participation: Gendered labor and collective rights paradigms in Mexico. *Gender & Society, 29*(6), 914–936.

Xekardaki A. et al. (2015) Neuropathological changes in aging brain. In P. Vlamos & A. Alexiou (Eds.), *GeNeDis 2014* (pp. 11–18). Advances in Experimental Medicine and Biology, 821. New York: Springer. doi: 10.1007/978–3–319–08939–3_6.

Yahalom, J. (2013). Mothers and the phenomenology of the memorable photograph. *Phenomenology & Practice, 7*(1), 126–138.

Yahalom, J. (2017). Levinasian caregiving: Dementia and the other-in-between. *Philosophy in the Contemporary World, 24*(1), 51–62.

Yarris, K. E. (2017). *Care across generations: Solidarity and sacrifice in transnational families*. Stanford, CA: Stanford University Press.

Yarris, K. E. (2014). "Pensando mucho" (thinking too much): Embodied distress among grandmothers in Nicaraguan transnational families. *Culture, Medicine, and Psychiatry, 38*(3), 473–498.

Young, J. C., & Garro, L. C. (1993). *Medical choice in a Mexican village*. Long Grove, IL: Waveland Press.

Young, K. (1976). *The social setting of migration: Factors affecting migration from a Sierra Zapotec village in Oaxaca, Mexico* (Unpublished doctoral dissertation). University of London, London, UK.

Index

incontinence, 85, 116–17, 140. *See also* bathing

India, 58, 70

indigenismo ideology, 9–11, 91, 175n11

Indigenous, as term, xv, 171n1

indigenous healers. See *curanderas*

indigenous psychology, 75–81, 188n8–9. See also *curanderas;* humoral medical theory

infectious diseases, 96

Instituto Nacional Indigenista (National Indigenous Institute), 90, 98

insurance systems, 55, 192n12

interdependency, 117–18, 156. *See also* family networks

intergenerational relationships, 4–5; Pablo and Vanessa on, 110–11; role reversal in, 112; of Sergio and Pedro, 35–36. *See also* family networks

irritability, 35, 72, 75, 110. *See also* anger

Isabelle, 39; on loneliness, 147; on Nicholas's condition and care, 86, 87, 91, 140

isolation. *See* loneliness

ixtli-in yollutl (face-heart), 188n8

Jackson, Michael, 68, 158

James, William, 24, 70, 77, 164

Japan, 58, 194n7

Jorge (age 20), 39

Jorge (age 70), 39, 92, 122

Juana, 39; care and support of, 61–64, 105; condition and symptoms of, 65–67, 72, 98–99

Juanita, 39, 50, 92, 122

Katzman, Robert, 185n22

Kearney, Michael, 14

khyâl (wind attacks), 22

Kleinman, Arthur, 21, 111, 113, 117

knowledge in medicine. *See* belief versus knowledge, medicinal

language: function of, 69–70, 187n1; interviews and theory on, 181n40. *See also* Spanish language; Zapotec language

Latour, Bruno, 25, 178n25

Laubscher, Leswin, 172n3

laughter, 68–69

Laura, 39; on caring for Leticia, 128; on Leticia's symptoms, 66, 115–16, 196n14

Leslie, Charles, 187n4

Leticia, 39; care and support of, 128, 196n14; condition and symptoms of, 66, 81, 115

Levinas, Emmanuel, xvi, 151–52, 173n2

Linda, 39, 53; on gossip, 150; on Pedro's diagnosis, 104; on Pedro's symptoms, 59, 68, 76, 122

"lived experience," 111–12, 193n1. *See also* phenomenology, as method

Lock, Margaret, 58

loneliness, 133, 137, 145–48, 151–55. *See also* depression; segre-social dynamics; social suffering

longevity rates, 46–47, 182nn9–11

Luis, 39, 66, 81

Lundbeck, 184n18

Luria, Alexander, 186n24

mal de ojo (evil eye), 73, 90

Manny, 72, 75–76

Manuel, 39; on family networks, 148; on gossip, 150; on Pedro's symptoms, 34, 35, 53, 58–59, 80, 122; work of, 40

Maria, 39; care and support of, 41, 108–10, 125–28; condition and symptoms of, 79, 100, 108, 124; hallucinations of, 124, 125; theft accusations by, 110,